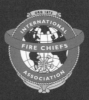

International Association of Fire Chiefs

EXAM PREP

Medical First Responder

By Dr. Ben A. Hirst,
Performance Training
Systems

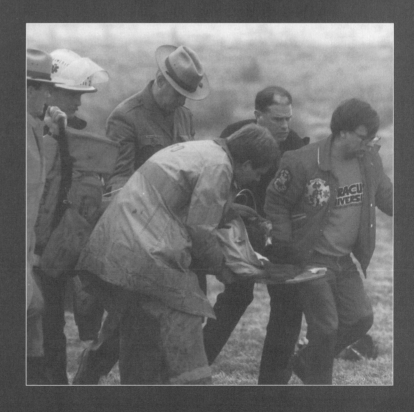

JONES AND BARTLETT PUBLISHERS
Sudbury, Massachusetts
BOSTON   TORONTO   LONDON   SINGAPORE

Jones and Bartlett Publishers
World Headquarters
40 Tall Pine Drive
Sudbury, MA 01776
978-443-5000
www.jbpub.com

Jones and Bartlett Publishers Canada
6339 Ormindale Way
Mississauga, Ontario L5V 1J2
Canada

Jones and Bartlett Publishers International
Barb House, Barb Mews
London W6 7PA
United Kingdom

International Association of Fire Chiefs
4025 Fair Ridge Drive
Fairfax, VA 22033
www.IAFC.org

Performance Training Systems, Inc.
760 U.S. Highway One, Suite 101
North Palm Beach, FL 33408
www.FireTestBanks.com

Jones and Bartlett's books and products are available through most bookstores and online booksellers. To contact Jones and Bartlett Publishers directly, call 800-832-0034, fax 978-443-8000, or visit our website www.jbpub.com.

Substantial discounts on bulk quantities of Jones and Bartlett's publications are available to corporations, professional associations, and other qualified organizations. For details and specific discount information, contact the special sales department at Jones and Bartlett via the above contact information or send an email to specialsales@jbpub.com.

Editorial Credits
Author: Dr. Ben A. Hirst

Production Credits
Chief Executive Officer: Clayton E. Jones
Chief Operating Officer: Donald W. Jones, Jr.
President, Higher Education and Professional Publishing: Robert W. Holland, Jr.
V.P., Sales and Marketing: William J. Kane
V.P., Production and Design: Anne Spencer
V.P., Manufacturing and Inventory Control: Therese Connell
Publisher, Public Safety Group: Kimberly Brophy

Editorial Assistant: Adrienne Zicht
Production Editor: Karen Ferreira
Director of Marketing: Alisha Weisman
Senior Photo Researcher: Kimberly Potvin
Cover Design: Kristin E. Ohlin
Interior Design: Anne Spencer
Composition: Northeast Compositors
Printing and Binding: Courier Stoughton

Copyright © 2006 by Jones and Bartlett Publishers, Inc. and Performance Training Systems, Inc.

Photo Credits
Cover photo © Craig Jackson/In the Dark Photography

ISBN-13: 978-0-7637-4214-0
ISBN-10: 0-7637-4214-7
6048

The procedures in this text are based on the most current recommendations of responsible sources. The publisher and Performance Training Systems, Inc. make no guarantees as to, and assume no responsibility for the correctness, sufficiency, or completeness of such information or recommendations. Other or additional safety measures may be required under particular circumstances. This text is intended solely as a guide to the appropriate procedures to be employed when responding to an emergency. It is not intended as a statement of the procedures required in any particular situation, because circumstances can vary widely from one emergency to another. Nor is it intended that this text shall in any way advise firefighting personnel concerning legal authority to perform the activities or procedures discussed. Such local determination should be made only with the aid of legal counsel.

Printed in the United States of America
10 09 08 07 06   10 9 8 7 6 5 4 3 2 1

CONTENTS

ACKNOWLEDGMENTS

More than nine paramedics have contributed to the development, validation, revision, and updating of the examination items included in this *Exam Prep* book. Their efforts are valued because of the credibility they provided. A special thanks goes to the recent Technical Review Committee for Medical First Responder for validating and updating the examination items to the latest DOT curriculum and latest publications: Deborah Estes, Pike Township, Indiana; Henry Michael Cantley, Arkansas Fire Academy, Arkansas; Scott Labadie, Palm Beach County Fire Rescue, Florida; Brenda P. Tenney, Connecticut Commission on Fire Prevention and Control, Connecticut; Walter Hirst, EMT-P, Delray Fire Department, Florida; Lt. Todd Lynch, EMT-P, Delray Fire Department, Florida; Ed Beardsley, EMT-P, Delray Fire Department, Florida; Chris Seay, EMT-P, Palm Beach County Fire Department, Florida. These individuals worked diligently to make considerable improvements in the examination items.

I want to thank my wife Elizabeth, my family, and friends who encouraged me to continue pressing forward with the work. Without their understanding and support, I would not have been able to meet the scheduled delivery date.

Last, but not least, I express my sincere thanks to my able staff: Ellen Korn, Administrative Assistant; Cristina Estrada, Sales Support; Paulette Kelly, Clerical Staff; Walter Hirst, Paramedic/Fire fighter and Director of Operations; Lt. Todd Lynch, Paramedic/Fire fighter and Regional Sales Manager; Chris Seay, Paramedic/Fire fighter and Regional Sales Manager; Ed Beardsley, Paramedic/Fire fighter and Regional Sales Manager. While I was away, in complete solitude, they kept the business going.

PREFACE

The Emergency Medical Service (EMS) is facing one of the most challenging periods in its history. Local, state, provincial, national, and international government organizations are under pressure to deliver ever-increasing services. The events of September 11, 2001, continued activities and threats by terrorist organizations worldwide, recent natural disasters, and the need to maximize available funds are part of the reason most EMS organizations are examining and reinventing their roles.

The challenge of reinventing the Emergency Medical Service to provide the first response efforts includes increasing professional requirements. Organizations such as the United States Department of Transportation, National Registry of Emergency Medical Technicians, and National Highway Traffic Safety Administration are having a dramatic influence on raising the professional qualifications of the first line of defense for emergency response. Most of the United States use training and testing materials developed and funded by these organizations as the basis for certification of Emergency Medical Service personnel.

Qualification standards have already been improved. Indeed, accreditation of training and certification are at the highest levels ever in the history of the Emergency Medical Service. These improvements are reflected in a better prepared first responder, but also have a noticeable effect on those individuals who serve. EMS providers are being required to expand their roles, acquire new knowledge, develop new and higher level technical skills, as well as participate in refresher and continuing education training programs on a regular basis.

The aftermath of September 11, along with several major natural disasters, has profoundly affected the Emergency Medical Service. Lessons learned, new technology, and the national focus on terrorism and weapons of mass destruction are placing much greater demands on emergency scene operations.

Emergency Medical Service personnel cannot afford to be complacent and continue to perform in the same way. Obvious dangers faced by first responders under current heightened security conditions require many adjustments in what is being taught to EMS personnel as they prepare to operate in an emergency environment. To meet this need, processes and modes of operation must be carefully examined and must be continuously monitored, changed, and updated.

The United States' national leaders constantly point to the first responders as our "first line of defense" against acts of terror and defense of life and property from extremely dangerous weapons that have never been used extensively in U.S. history. Several major disasters such as hurricanes, tornadoes, wildland fires, flooding, major injury incidents, and earthquakes have raised the awareness of planners, first responders, and hospitals regarding their response and mediation capabilities.

Some Emergency Medical Service programs are steeped in tradition. Nevertheless, it is critical that we question our traditions and our thinking to bring our knowledge, skills, and abilities in line with the demands of today's real world.

Many things have been learned from the September 11 attack on America. Some of these lessons learned were the result of our reluctance to change processes and procedures (i.e. our traditions). As great as our traditions are, members of the Emergency Medical

EXAM PREP: MEDICAL FIRST RESPONDER

Service industry must not stop reflecting on the paramount reasons for our existence—namely, to provide quality care, save lives, and perform our tasks with personal safety as the number one concern. These are very important reasons to exist, to continuously improve, and to move from a good Emergency Medical Service industry to a great Emergency Medical Service industry.

A few words about knowing vital strategic and tactical information are in order. Many organizations focus a great deal of their training time and effort on the performance side of EMS. That is essential and is the bottom line for developing skilled medical first responders. The dark side of this approach to training is that it fails to emphasize key knowledge requirements. Often, it is not what we did or didn't do as medical first responders, but what we could have done if we had a strong base of knowledge that helps to analyze and detect a need for action outside our routine tasks. How many times does Plan A go wrong at the emergency scene? How well do we transition from Plan A to Plan B or Plan C? Are our emergency incident communications adequate, timely, precise, and getting to the right people? These questions may never be answered, but they do require the Emergency Medical Service as a whole, and each responder in particular, to focus equally on the knowledge portion of emergency responses to help improve the performance side of our tasks.

Pre-planning for an emergency target hazard is important; knowing what can go wrong is essential. Knowledge is the potential power we must acquire to make important adjustments during the emergency incident, to continuously size up the situation, and to alter our plan of action as needed and required.

Our supervisors, responders, and support personnel must develop a solid knowledge base so that better judgments, sizeups, and emergency actions can be decided and implemented. Research in education and training over the years has concluded that lack of knowledge is one of the key reasons why tasks are not performed, poorly performed, or performed in a manner that did not achieve the expected results.

Hazardous materials are everywhere in the American society. Homes contain hazardous materials, as do businesses, warehouses, places of public assembly, and almost every other type of structure. They can be found in open areas like farm land, wooded areas where clandestine labs operate, and countless other outdoor areas. The first responders must learn to treat fires, collapses, and even traffic accidents as probable hazardous materials incidents. Personal safety at the emergency scene must be the primary focus.

There is a great deal to learn and master regarding the nine hazard classes identified and described by the United States Department of Transportation (DOT). Many hazardous materials incidents occur in the United States every day. First responders must realize that their safety and the safety of citizens are paramount during the response to a hazardous materials incident. We all know that responder safety is always the first priority during incident operations. This realization is extremely critical when hazardous materials are detected or the preincident plan suggests that they are present. Proactive planning can aid the first responder to handle critical hazardous materials incidents efficiently and effectively. One of the most harmful situations is to discover a hazardous materials incident well into the response situation. The unexpected often causes undue exposure to harmful substances that can result in immediate and long-term health effects. The first responder and the initial hazardous materials operations crew must have highly developed recognition skills, identification skills, and must know the isolation and protection parameters required for the incident.

In the recent history of the EMS, it has become abundantly clear that learning is a careerlong, lifelong requirement that serves as the foundation for the demands that lie ahead. Members of the EMS must adopt this principle to move from a tradition-rich past to become truly great providers and protectors available to everyone we serve. We cannot correct the mistakes of the past, but we can use lessons learned to prevent similar mistakes in the future. Knowledge is power. Efficient and effective people are the solution to moving from a good Emergency Medical Service to a truly great one.

In the past 18 years, Performance Training Systems, Inc. (PTS) has emerged as the leading provider of valid testing materials for certification, promotion, and training for Fire and Emergency Medical Service personnel. More than 35 test-item banks, containing more than 22,000 questions, provide the basis for the validated examinations. All products are based on the NFPA Professional Qualifications Standards and selected parts of the DOT's National Standard Curriculum for Medical First Responders.

Over the past eight years, PTS has conducted research supporting the development of the Systematic Approach to Examination Preparation® (SAEP). SAEP has resulted in consistent improvement in scores for persons taking certification, promotion, and training completion examinations. This *Exam Prep* manual is designed to assist medical first responders improve their knowledge, skills, and abilities while seeking training program completion, certification, and promotion. Using the features of SAEP, coupled with helpful examination-taking tips and hints, will help ensure improved performance from a more knowledgeable and skilled medical first responder

All examination questions used in SAEP were written by medical first responders. Technical content has been validated through the use of current technical textbooks and other technical reference materials; and job content has been validated by the use of technical review committees representative of the medical first responder profession and representatives of training and certification organizations. The examination questions in this *Exam Prep* manual represent an approximate 50 percent sample of the *Medical First Responder Test-Item Bank* developed and maintained by PTS. These testing materials and 33 other test-item banks are being used by 69 fire service certification agencies worldwide, 126 fire academies, and more than 340 fire department training divisions. Forty-six of the fifty state certification agencies use these testing materials in their certification programs.

Purposes of the Emergency Medical *Exam Prep* Manuals

Performance Training Systems, Inc. provides *Exam Prep* manuals for the following EMS levels:

- Medical First Responder
- Emergency Medical Technician—Basic
- Emergency Medical Technician—Paramedic

The Emergency Medical *Exam Prep* manuals are designed to provide a random sample of examination items from the major sections of the DOT's National Standard Curriculum. Each examination is designed specifically to help you prepare for your national examination and your local state certification or refresher examination. The *Exam Prep* manuals can also be used in initial training programs and for refresher training.

Since the examination questions have been job-content validated using groups of expert judges from the job incumbent categories, they may also be used for preparing for promotional examinations and for employee selection examinations as long as the pool of job candidates have completed appropriate training and certification in the EMS technical level. The *Exam Prep* manuals are not intended for use in selecting individuals from the general public who have not had appropriate EMS training and certification. Contact Performance Training Systems, Inc for specific information and procedures on using the *Exam Prep* manuals for employee selection or promotion.

Emergency Medical Service members generally don't like to take examinations. For that matter, few people really like them. The primary purposes of the *Exam Prep* series are to help EMS personnel develop an improved level of knowledge, eliminate examination-taking fear, build self-confidence, and develop good study and information mastery skills. For more information on the number of available test-item banks and the processes of development and validation, visit *medictestbanks.com*.

Introduction to the Systematic Approach to Examination Preparation

How does SAEP work? SAEP is an organized process of carefully researched phases that permits each person to proceed through examination preparation at that individual's own pace. At certain points, self-study is required to move from one phase of the program to another. Receiving and then using feedback on one's progress is the basis of SAEP. It is important to follow the program steps carefully to realize the full benefits of the system.

SAEP allows you to prepare carefully for your next comprehensive training, promotional, or certification examination. Just follow the steps to success. PTS, the leader in producing promotional and certification examinations for the Fire and Emergency Medical Service industry for more than 18 years, has both the experience and the testing expertise to help you meet your professional goals.

Using the *Exam Prep* manual will enable you to pinpoint areas of weakness in terms of first responder requirements, and the feedback will provide the reference and page numbers to help you research the questions that you miss or guess using current technical reference materials. This program comprises a three-examination set for Medical First Responder as described in the selected parts of the DOT's National Standard Curriculum.

Primary benefits of SAEP in preparing for these examinations include the following:

- Emphasis on areas of weakness
- Immediate feedback
- Savings in time and energy
- Learning technical material through context and association
- Helpful examination preparation practices and hints

Phases of SAEP

SAEP is organized in three distinct phases for Medical First Responder as described in portions of the DOT's National Standard Curriculum. These phases are briefly described next.

Phase I

Phase I includes three examinations containing items that are selected from each major part of the DOT's National Standard Curriculum. An essential part of the SAEP design is to survey your present level of knowledge and build on it for subsequent examination and self-directed study activities. Therefore, it is suggested that you read the reference materials, but do not study or look up any answers while taking the initial examination. Upon completion of the initial examination, you will complete a feedback activity and record examination-items that you missed or that you guessed. We ask you to perform certain tasks during the feedback activity. Once you have completed the initial examination and have researched the answers for any questions you missed, you may proceed to the next examination. This process is repeated through and including the third examination in the Medical First Responder series, depending on the level of qualification you are seeking.

Phase II

Phase II contains important information about examination-item construction. It provides insight regarding the examination-item developers, the way in which they apply their technology, and hints and tips to help you score higher on any examination. Make sure you read this phase carefully. It is a good practice to read it twice, and study the information a day or two prior to your scheduled examination.

Phase III

Phase III information addresses the mental and physical aspects of examination preparation. By all means, do not skip this part of your preparation. Points can be lost if you are not ready—both physically and mentally—for the examination. If you have participated in sporting or other competitive events, you know the importance of this level of preparation. There is no substitute for readiness. Just being able to answer the questions will not help you achieve a level of excellence and move you to the top of the examination list for training, promotion, or certification. Quality preparation involves much more than simply answering examination items.

Supplemental Practice Examination Program

The supplemental practice examination program differs from the SAEP program in several ways. First, it is provided over the Internet 24 hours a day, 7 days a week. In addition, this supplemental practice examination allows you to make final preparations immediately before your examination date. You will receive an immediate feedback report that includes the questions missed and the references and page numbers pertaining to those missed questions. The practice examination can help you concentrate on your areas of greatest weakness and will save you time and energy immediately before the examination date. If you choose this method of preparation, do not "cram" for the examination. The upcoming helpful hints for examination preparation will explain the reasons for avoiding a "cramming exercise." A supplemental practice examination is available with the purchase of this *Exam Prep* manual by using the enclosed registration form. Do not forget to fax a copy of your Personal Progress Plotter along with your registration form. The data supplied on your Personal Progress Plotter will be kept confidential and will be used by PTS to make future improvements in the *Exam Prep* series. You may take a short practice examination to get the procedure clear in your mind by going to *www.webtesting.cc*.

Good luck in your efforts to improve your knowledge and skills. Our primary goal is to improve the Emergency Medical Service one person at a time. We want your feedback and impressions of the system to help us implement improvements in future editions of the *Exam Prep* series of books. Address your comments and suggestions to *www.medictestbanks.com*.

--- Rule 1 ---

Examination preparation is not easy. Preparation is 95% perspiration and 5% inspiration.

--- Rule 2 ---

Follow the steps very carefully. Do not try to reinvent or shortcut the system. It really works just as it was designed to!

Personal Progress Plotter

Medical First Responder Exam Prep

Name: ——————————————————

Date Started: ——————————————————

Date Completed: ——————————————————

Medical First Responder	Number Guessed	Number Missed	Examination Score
Examination I-1			
Examination I-2			
Examination I-3			

Formula to compute Examination Score = ((Number guessed + Number missed) X Point Value per examination item) subtracted from 100

Note: 150-item examination = 0.67 points per examination item
100-item examination = 1.0 point per examination item

Example: In Examination I-1 or I-2, 5 examination items were guessed and 8 were missed, for a total of 13 on a 100-item examination. The examination score would be 100 − (13 × 1.0 Points) = 87.0

Example: In Examination I-3, 5 examination items were guessed and 8 were missed, for a total of 13 on a 150-item examination. The examination score would be 150 − (13 × 0.67 Points) = 91.3

Note: To receive your free online practice examination, you must fax a copy of your completed Personal Progress Plotter along with your registration form.

PHASE I

Medical First Responder

Examination I-1, Beginning DOT National Standard Curriculum for Medical First Responders

Examination I-1 contains 100 examination items. Read the reference materials but do not study prior to taking the examination. The examination is designed to identify your weakest areas in terms of selected parts of the DOT's National Standard Curriculum. Some steps in SAEP will require self-study of specific reference materials. Remove Examination I-1 from the book. Mark all answers in ink to ensure that no changes are made later. Do not mark through answers or change answers in any way once you have selected your answers.

 Step 1—Take Examination I-1. When you have completed Examination I-1, go to Appendix A and compare your answers with the correct answers. Each answer identifies reference materials with the relevant page numbers. If you missed the answer to the examination item, you have a source for conducting your correct answer research.

 Step 2—Score Examination I-1. How many examination items did you miss? Write the number of missed examination items in the blank in ink _____. Enter the number of examination items you guessed in this blank _____. Enter these numbers in the designated locations on your Personal Progress Plotter.

 Step 3—Now the learning begins! Carefully research the page cited in the reference material for the correct answer. For instance, use Jones and Bartlett, AAOS, *First Responder, Your First Response in Emergency Care*, Third Edition, go to the page number provided and find the answer.

—————————— Rule 3 ——————————

Mark with an "X" any examination items for which you guessed the answer. For maximum return on effort, you should also research any answer that you guessed even if you guessed correctly. Find the correct answer, highlight it, and then read the entire paragraph that contains the answer. Be honest and mark all questions on which you guessed. Some examinations have a correction for guessing built into the scoring process. The correction for guessing can reduce your final examination score. If you are guessing, you are not mastering the material.

——————— **Rule 4** ———————

Read questions twice if you have any misunderstanding, especially if the question contains complex directions or activities.

——————— **Helpful Hint** ———————

Most of the time your first impression is the best. More than 41% of changed answers during PTS's SAEP field test were changed from a right answer to a wrong answer. Another 33% were changed from one wrong answer to another wrong answer. Only 26% of answers were changed from wrong to right. In fact, three participants did not make a perfect score of 100% because they changed one right answer to a wrong one! Think twice before you change your answer. The odds are not in your favor.

——————— **Helpful Hint** ———————

Researching correct answers is one of the most important activities in SAEP. Locate the correct answer for all missed examination items. Highlight the correct answer. Then read the entire paragraph containing the answer. This will put the answer in context for you and provide important learning by association.

——————— **Helpful Hint** ———————

Proceed through all missed examination items using the same technique. Reading the entire paragraph improves retention of the information and helps you develop an association with the material and learn the correct answers. This step may sound simple. A major finding during the development and field testing of SAEP was that you learn from your mistakes.

Examination I-1

Directions

Remove Examination I-1 from the manual. First, take a careful look at the examination. There should be 100 examination items. Notice that a blank line precedes each examination item number. This line is provided for you to enter the answer to the examination item. Write the answer in ink. Remember the rule about not changing your answers. Our research has shown that changed answers are often incorrect, and, more often than not, the answer that is chosen first is correct.

If you guess the answer to a question, place an "X" or a check mark by your answer. This step is vitally important as you gain and master knowledge. We will explain how we treat the "guessed" items later in SAEP.

Take the examination. Once you complete it, go to Appendix A and score your examination. Once the examination is scored, carefully follow the directions for feedback on the missed and guessed examination items.

_____ **1.** All of the following tools can be used to help unlock a vehicle door **except** a:
   A. slim-jim.
   B. screwdriver.
   C. wire hook.
   D. K Tool.

_____ **2.** The **first** thing you should do when you come upon a vehicle that is overturned or on its side is to:
   A. gain access through a window.
   B. turn the vehicle right side up.
   C. stabilize the vehicle.
   D. pull the occupants through the rear window.

_____ **3.** Always feel the _____ of the door before opening it when fire is suspected on the other side.
   A. bottom
   B. top
   C. door knob
   D. door jamb

_____ **4.** If you suspect a gas leak, **do not**:
   A. use the doorbell.
   B. transmit on your radio.
   C. turn on/off the lights.
   D. do all of the above.

_____ **5.** Remove patients from a vehicle **only** when:
   A. life saving care is required.
   B. the patient is having an anxiety attack.
   C. they would be more comfortable in your vehicle.
   D. there is severe weather approaching.

_____ **6.** Which of the following **is not** a part of the upper respiratory system?
   A. Alveoli
   B. Nasopharynx
   C. Oropharynx
   D. Larynx
   E. Epiglottis

_____ **7.** The _____ is a tubular structure that begins below the vocal cords and extends into the chest and carries air into and out of the lungs.
   A. bronchi
   B. alveoli
   C. trachea
   D. epiglottis
   E. bronchioles

_____ **8.** The _____ are small sacs at the end of the respiratory system where the exchange of gases occurs with the bloodstream.
   A. bronchioles
   B. bronchi
   C. cilia
   D. alveoli
   E. vocal cords

_____ **9.** The **best** method of opening the airway in patients who have suffered, or potentially suffered, a traumatic injury is:
   A. the head tilt–chin lift method.
   B. the jaw thrust.
   C. the nasopharyngeal method.
   D. Any of the above methods may be used.

_____ **10.** Suctioning should be performed for no longer than _____ seconds in adult patients.
   A. 5
   B. 10
   C. 15
   D. 20
   E. 25

_____ **11.** An acceptable tool for first responders to use in ventilating a patient is:
   A. a pocket mask.
   B. an intubation kit.
   C. a bag-valve-mask device.
   D. Both A and C.

_____ **12.** The bag-valve-mask device is **most effective** when:
   A. used by two first responders.
   B. used in conjunction with a pocket mask.
   C. used on pediatric patients only.
   D. used without the mask portion.
   E. patients are breathing on their own.

_____ 13. The _____ is an airway adjunct device that is a flexible rubber or plastic tube designed to be inserted into the nose and extend to the back of the pharynx.
A. oropharyngeal airway
B. endotracheal tube
C. nasopharyngeal airway
D. suction catheter
E. nonrebreathing mask

_____ 14. The _____ provides the patient with the highest level of oxygen without performing advanced life support airway procedures.
A. nasal cannula
B. oropharyngeal airway
C. suction catheter
D. nonrebreathing mask
E. nasopharyngeal airway

_____ 15. The proper oxygen flow rate when using a nonrebreathing mask is:
A. 1 liter per minute.
B. 2–4 liters per minute.
C. 10–15 liters per minute.
D. 20–25 liters per minute.
E. 35 liters per minute.

_____ 16. The **only** artery that carries unoxygenated blood away from the heart is called the:
A. coronary arteriole.
B. hepatic artery.
C. pulmonary artery.
D. aorta.

_____ 17. To provide proper circulatory function, a typical adult must maintain a volume of _____ liters of blood.
A. 5–6
B. 7–8
C. 3–4
D. 9–10

_____ 18. The **quickest** and **most effective** way of controlling most forms of bleeding is by applying:
A. ice packs.
B. a tourniquet.
C. direct pressure.
D. a band-aid.

_____ 19. You **should not** use elevation in combination with direct pressure when dealing with:
A. the amputation of an extremity.
B. a possible extremity fracture.
C. muscle lesions.
D. a pelvic fracture.

_____ **20.** There are 22 major pressure point sites used to control bleeding (11 sites on each side of the body). Which two sites are commonly part of a first responder's training?
   A. Carotid
   B. Carpel pedal
   C. Brachial and femoral
   D. Radial

_____ **21.** Which of the following **is not** a treatment a first responder provides for external bleeding?
   A. Applying heat packs to the injury site
   B. Direct pressure to the site of the bleeding
   C. Elevation of the injured extremity
   D. Use of pressure points
   E. Applying sterile dressings or bandages

_____ **22.** An internal injury causing blood vessels and organs to be crushed or ruptured by a severe blow to the body, but with no cuts to the skin is a type of:
   A. systemic laceration.
   B. avulsion.
   C. penetrating trauma.
   D. blunt trauma.

_____ **23.** A wound ranging from a simple scrape to a tearing of the skin is called a/an:
   A. fibrous wound.
   B. closed wound.
   C. open wound.
   D. bruise.

_____ **24.** A fertilized egg is an embryo until it reaches the eighth week, then it is called a/an:
   A. uterus.
   B. placenta.
   C. womb.
   D. fetus.

_____ **25.** The development period of a fetus is divided into 3-month segments called:
   A. semesters.
   B. trimonths.
   C. trimesters.
   D. trisegments.

_____ **26.** Labor pains normally come at regular intervals and last for about:
   A. 2 to 3 minutes.
   B. 30 seconds to 1 minute.
   C. 30 minutes to 1 hour.
   D. 3 to 4 minutes.

_____ **27.** The time from the start of one contraction to the beginning of the next
    is called:
    A. false labor/Braxton Hicks.
    B. refractory period.
    C. interval time.
    D. contraction time.

_____ **28.** Placement of sheets or towels for a mother preparing for delivery include all of
    the following **except**:
    A. one under the mother's buttocks.
    B. one under the mother's head.
    C. one under the mother's vaginal opening.
    D. one over the mother's abdomen.

_____ **29.** Consider a birth delivery to be normal if:
    A. it lasts only five minutes.
    B. the baby's head appears first.
    C. the feet present first.
    D. the shoulders appear first.

_____ **30.** In an unresponsive patient, the first three steps to determine the presence of
    spontaneous respirations are:
    A. shake, shout, feel.
    B. poke, pinch, prod.
    C. reach, rub, retract.
    D. look, listen, feel.

_____ **31.** Which of the following **is not** an early part of the chain of survival for victims
    of cardiac arrest?
    A. CPR
    B. Defibrillation
    C. Advanced cardiac life support (ACLS)
    D. Electrocardiogram interpretation
    E. Access

_____ **32.** A/An _____ External Defibrillator unit, once attached to a patient,
    requires the provider to initiate the defibrillation of a patient if a shockable
    rhythm is determined to be present.
    A. Automatic
    B. Stationary
    C. Non-automatic
    D. Semi-automatic

_____ **33.** Which of the following statements about AEDs **is false**?
    A. AEDs require the user to interpret the cardiac rhythm.
    B. AEDs should be inspected regularly.
    C. First responders should check the batteries on the AED unit per the
        manufacturer's recommendations.
    D. AED pouches often carry extra supplies like razors and gauze.
    E. Some AEDs have a screen that displays the heart rhythm.

_____ **34.** In _____ the electrical and mechanical activities of the heart have stopped.
  A. ventricular fibrillation
  B. atrial tachycardia
  C. asystole
  D. ventricular tachycardia
  E. regular sinus rhythm

_____ **35.** In which of the following situations can an AED be used?
  A. A conscious patient experiencing trouble breathing
  B. A patient in cardiac arrest
  C. An unconscious child who has a pulse
  D. A conscious adult having chest pain
  E. All of the above.

_____ **36.** Which of the following is a description of the correct placement for AED electrodes?
  A. Under the right clavicle and over the lower left rib cage
  B. Under the right clavicle and on the patient's stomach
  C. On the sternum and over the lower left rib cage
  D. Over the right lower rib cage and over the left lower rib cage
  E. Any of the above will work. Placement of the AED electrodes is not important.

_____ **37.** Which of the statements about using an AED is **true**?
  A. While the AED is analyzing the patient's rhythm, it is acceptable to be touching the patient or continue performing CPR.
  B. The AED will ask the user to interpret the heart rhythm.
  C. CPR must be stopped for the entire cycle of analysis for the AED to accurately assess the patient's heart rhythm.
  D. Local protocols are not important to the first responder regarding the use of AEDs.
  E. First responders should immediately attach an AED to every patient.

_____ **38.** If a patient in cardiac arrest is found with a bulge in the chest thought to be an artificial pacemaker, the first responder should:
  A. place the AED electrode directly on top of the bulge in the chest.
  B. place the AED electrode to the left of the bulge and several inches lower (toward the feet).
  C. place both AED electrodes on the lower left ribcage area.
  D. discontinue use of the AED.
  E. place the AED electrode on the shoulder above the bulge.

_____ **39.** _____ are the pads in contact with a patient's skin that allow electrical impulses to be read by a heart monitor, and allow the delivery of an electrical defibrillation if necessary.
  A. Dysrhythmias
  B. Electrodes
  C. Electrocardiograms
  D. Contraindications
  E. Medication patches

_____ **40.** Available oxygen is used up in about _____ minutes after the heart
stops beating.
  A. four to six
  B. one
  C. two to four
  D. three to five

_____ **41.** A patient who is lying face up on the ground is in a _____ position.
  A. supine
  B. prone
  C. proximal
  D. distal
  E. medial

_____ **42.** The front of the body is referred to as:
  A. posterior.
  B. medial.
  C. proximal.
  D. anterior.
  E. distal.

_____ **43.** The human brain is housed and protected by the:
  A. vertebrae.
  B. coccyx.
  C. skull/cranial cavity.
  D. fontanels.

_____ **44.** When performing a detailed physical exam, the first responder should divide
the abdomen into _____ and palpate each individually.
  A. two halves
  B. three sections
  C. four quadrants
  D. six sections
  E. eight sections

_____ **45.** The <u>lowest</u> point on the sternum, which is used as a landmark for locating
proper hand position during cardiopulmonary resuscitation (CPR), is the:
  A. coccyx.
  B. fontanel.
  C. xiphoid process.
  D. thorax.
  E. diaphragm.

_____ **46.** The muscle that separates the thoracic and abdominal cavities is the:
  A. pectorals.
  B. xiphoid process.
  C. trapezius.
  D. thorax.
  E. diaphragm.

_____ **47.** The three main components of the circulatory system are the _____, the blood vessels, and the blood.
A. aorta
B. stomach
C. heart
D. coronary arteries
E. pancreas

_____ **48.** At times, a first responder will be unable to determine the age of an infant or child; therefore, an estimate of age can be determined based on all of the following **except**:
A. physical size.
B. level of consciousness.
C. emotional responses.
D. interaction with the first responder.
E. language skills.

_____ **49.** When infants and small children suffer from a head injury that presents with shock, you should also suspect:
A. child abuse.
B. thermal burns.
C. an extremity fracture.
D. internal injuries.

_____ **50.** Children are more vulnerable to _____ than adults because of their larger and heavier head and of their under-developed neck muscles and bone structures.
A. scalp wounds
B. eye injuries
C. spinal injuries
D. seizures

_____ **51.** If a suspected hip or pelvis injury has occurred in a child, you should do all of the following **except**:
A. monitor vital signs for shock.
B. rock the hips to check for instability.
C. check for bleeding or bloody discharge from the genital area.
D. arrange for transport as soon as possible.

_____ **52.** The extent of medical procedures a first responder is authorized to perform is called the:
A. medical release.
B. scope of practice/care.
C. duty to act.
D. physician relationship.
E. skill set.

_____ **53.** It **is** **not** a role of a first responder to:
    A. act as liaison with other types of response and professional agencies.
    B. gather important information.
    C. handle safety.
    D. provide advanced life support skills.
    E. provide emergency care to patients based on findings in a patient assessment.

_____ **54.** Which of the following **is** **not** an organizational element of an emergency medical service (EMS) system?
    A. Resource management
    B. Transportation
    C. Rehabilitation
    D. Communication
    E. Public information and education

_____ **55.** The United States Department of Transportation (DOT) develops curricula for _____ different levels of emergency medical service providers.
    A. 10
    B. 8
    C. 6
    D. 5
    E. 4

_____ **56.** _____ are designed to deal with life threatening injuries and have surgeons on hand for immediate surgical intervention.
    A. Burn centers
    B. Poison centers
    C. Trauma centers
    D. Prenatal centers

_____ **57.** _____ is a formal relationship between the emergency medical service providers and the physician responsible for out-of-hospital emergency medical care.
    A. Medical monitoring
    B. Health care tracking
    C. Provider monitoring
    D. Medical oversight
    E. Physician tracking

_____ **58.** What kind of medical control occurs when no direct contact is made with a physician in the course of treating a patient?
    A. Indirect (off-line) medical control
    B. Inherent medical control
    C. Direct (online) medical control
    D. Intermediate medical control
    E. Online medical control

Portland Community College

_____ **59.** In order to expose a gunshot or knife wound, the first responder should avoid disturbing evidence such as:
  A. bloodstains.
  B. suicide notes.
  C. tire marks.
  D. holes in clothing.

_____ **60.** _____ is the voluntary agreement by a patient to receive emergency medical treatment.
  A. Consent
  B. Abandonment
  C. Scope of practice
  D. Liability
  E. Competence

_____ **61.** A patient who is awake and alert and who verbalizes her consent for the first responder to provide care has given:
  A. implied consent.
  B. express consent.
  C. emancipated consent.
  D. competent consent.
  E. inherent consent.

_____ **62.** A patient who is unconscious provides a first responder:
  A. implied consent.
  B. express consent.
  C. emancipated consent.
  D. competent consent.
  E. inherent consent.

_____ **63.** What term describes the ability of a patient to understand questions, act responsibly, and comprehend the implications of decisions?
  A. Consent
  B. Emancipation
  C. Liability
  D. Competence
  E. Causation

_____ **64.** A first responder who inappropriately leaves a patient without having been relieved of patient care responsibility may be guilty of:
  A. emancipation.
  B. express consent.
  C. breaching.
  D. damages.
  E. abandonment.

_____ **65.** _____ is a deviation from the accepted standard of care resulting in further injury to a patient.
A. Abandonment
B. Breaching
C. Causation
D. Liability
E. Negligence

_____ **66.** When lifting patients, keep the back _____ and use the muscles in the _____.
A. bent; legs
B. straight; legs
C. straight; arms
D. straight; stomach
E. bent; arms

_____ **67.** When lifting an object or patient, keep the weight being lifted:
A. as close to the body as possible.
B. as far away from the body as possible.
C. to the left side of the body.
D. to the right side of the body.

_____ **68.** When lifting a patient, stand with your feet:
A. 3 feet apart.
B. together.
C. shoulder-width apart.
D. one in front of the other.

_____ **69.** Which of the following **is** a lifting and moving device used in emergency medical services?
A. Wheeled stretcher
B. Stair chair
C. Scoop (or orthopedic) stretcher
D. Backboard
E. All of the above.

_____ **70.** The term for the position a patient assumes to compensate for pain and discomfort is:
A. position of comfort.
B. recovery positioning.
C. urgent positioning.
D. indicated position.
E. position of patient care.

_____ **71.** When first responders move a trauma or non-trauma patient after stabilization and mitigation of immediate dangers, it is considered a/an _____ move.
A. urgent
B. position of comfort
C. nonurgent/nonemergency
D. immediate danger
E. intermediate

_____ **72.** _____ is/are sudden, involuntary contractions of a group of muscles
caused by a disturbance in brain function.
A. Fevers
B. Hypoxia
C. Seizures
D. Posticals

_____ **73.** A heart attack is caused when a _____ is occluded and a portion of the
heart is deprived of blood supply and oxygen.
A. coronary artery
B. superior vena cava
C. brachial artery
D. radial artery
E. right atrium

_____ **74.** _____ is a condition where the body is exposed to a cold environment
and is unable to compensate for the heat loss, resulting in an abnormally low
core temperature.
A. Heat exhaustion
B. Hypothermia
C. Heatstroke
D. Hyperthermia
E. Frostbite

_____ **75.** Which of the following **is not** a potential sign or symptom of a local
cold emergency?
A. Bright red skin color
B. Loss of feeling or sensation in the affected area
C. Swelling
D. Blisters
E. Pain or numbness in the affected area

_____ **76.** Which of the following statements is **false** regarding the treatment of a patient
with hypothermia and/or a local cold emergency?
A. Attempt to break any blisters present.
B. Refrain from rubbing or massaging injury or area involved.
C. Do not apply heat to deep cold injuries.
D. Refrain from allowing a patient to walk on an affected extremity.
E. Handle patients very gently.

_____ **77.** Which of the following is a sign or symptom of a patient experiencing
anaphylactic shock?
A. Hives
B. Difficulty breathing
C. Swelling of the face, lips, or tongue
D. Cyanosis
E. All of the above.

_____ **78.** Which of the following **is not** one of the four methods of allergen/poison exposure?
   A. Injection
   B. Insertion
   C. Ingestion
   D. Inhalation
   E. Absorption

_____ **79.** Which of the following is the life-threatening third stage of heat exposure where body systems begin to shut down?
   A. Heat seizures
   B. Heat cramps
   C. Heatstroke
   D. Heat exhaustion
   E. Hypothermia

_____ **80.** _____ is a system used to prioritize patients based on severity of injury and survivability.
   A. MCI management
   B. Incident Management System (IMS)
   C. Placards
   D. Triage
   E. Accountability

_____ **81.** Injuries to the _____ are often associated with head injuries.
   A. trachea
   B. spine/neck
   C. orbit
   D. maxilla

_____ **82.** All of the following are signs and symptoms of a brain injury **except**:
   A. bleeding or fluid from the ears.
   B. loss of consciousness.
   C. pupils that are unequal, slow or non-reactive to light.
   D. chest pain.

_____ **83.** An injury that causes blood vessels to rupture in the brain is called a/an:
   A. avulsion.
   B. concussion.
   C. laceration.
   D. contusion.

_____ **84.** The head, spinal column, and chest make up the:
   A. maxilla skeleton.
   B. midline.
   C. axial skeleton.
   D. cranium.

_____ **85.** Which component of the nervous system contains the brain and spinal cord?
   A. The central nervous system
   B. The main nervous system
   C. The peripheral nervous system
   D. The autonomic system
   E. The sensory nervous system

_____ **86.** Upper extremity injuries should be splinted with the hand:
   A. higher than the heart.
   B. palm up.
   C. in the position of function.
   D. across the chest.

_____ **87.** When dealing with suspected extremity dislocation, it is important to remember to:
   A. splint in the position found.
   B. apply manual traction.
   C. attempt to reduce it in the field.
   D. return to the position of function.

_____ **88.** Possible complications of extremity fractures include which of the following?
   A. Internal bleeding
   B. Restricted blood flow
   C. Soft tissue damage
   D. All of the above.

_____ **89.** When a first responder gathers patient information to determine the nature of an illness or injury including interviews and physical examination, this is called:
   A. patient assessment.
   B. secondary survey.
   C. nature of illness.
   D. mechanism of injury.

_____ **90.** Patients are cared for on the scene based on:
   A. diagnosis.
   B. bystander information.
   C. mechanism of injury.
   D. signs and symptoms.

_____ **91.** The components of patient assessment should include all of the following **except**:
   A. first responder safety.
   B. determining the level of patient's responsiveness.
   C. estimated transport time.
   D. patient safety.

_____ **92.** A force(s) that may have caused injury is called:
  A. trauma protocol.
  B. nature of illness.
  C. mechanism of injury.
  D. gravitational prolapse.

_____ **93.** Part of a patient assessment designed to detect and correct life threatening problems is called:
  A. rapid trauma assessment.
  B. secondary survey.
  C. initial assessment.
  D. tertiary assessment.

_____ **94.** The ABCs of emergency care stand for all of the following **except**:
  A. breathing.
  B. alertness.
  C. circulation.
  D. airway.

_____ **95.** Situations that puts you, patients, and bystanders in danger are called:
  A. emergencies.
  B. wreckage.
  C. hazards.
  D. alarms.

_____ **96.** First responders will be granted protection from civil liability if, while acting in good faith, they provide care to the level of training to the **best** of their ability under the:
  A. Good Samaritan Law.
  B. Davis Act.
  C. Hold No Harm Statute.
  D. Myers Act.

_____ **97.** Which of the following **is not** a way to combat stress?
  A. Eating a healthy diet
  B. Regular exercise
  C. Isolation
  D. Elimination or limitation of alcohol consumption
  E. Meditation

_____ **98.** Which of the following is a warning sign of stress?
  A. Isolation
  B. Loss of appetite
  C. Problems sleeping
  D. Anxiety
  E. All of the above.

_____ **99.** The five stages of the grieving process are denial, _____, bargaining, depression, and acceptance.
  A. solitude
  B. anxiety
  C. anger
  D. isolation
  E. annoyance

_____**100.** In the _____ phase of the grieving process, a person may refuse to accept the death or dying process.
  A. anger
  B. denial
  C. depression
  D. solitude
  E. acceptance

Did you score higher than 80 percent on Examination I-1? Circle Yes or No in ink. (We will return to your answer to this question later in SAEP).

Now that you have finished the Feedback Step for Examination I-1, it is time to repeat the process by taking another comprehensive examination of the *DOT, First Responder National Standard Curriculum.*

Examination I-2, Adding Difficulty and Depth

During Examination I-2 progress will be made in developing depth of knowledge and skills.

Step 1—Take Examination I-2. When you have completed Examination I-2, go to Appendix A and compare your answers with the correct answers.

Step 2—Score Examination I-2. How many examination items did you miss? Write the number of missed examination items in the blank in ink _____. Enter the number of examination items you guessed in this blank _____. Enter these numbers in the designated locations on your Personal Progress Plotter.

Step 3—Once again, the learning begins. During the feedback step, research the correct answer using the Appendix A information for Examination I-2. Highlight the correct answer during your research of the reference materials. Read the entire paragraph containing the correct answer.

— Helpful Hint —

Follow each step carefully to realize the best return on effort. Would you consider investing your money in a venture without some chance of earning a return on that investment? Examination preparation is no different. You are investing time and expecting a significant return for that time. If, indeed, time is money, then you are investing money and are due a return on that investment. Doing things right and doing the right things in examination preparation will ensure the maximum return on effort.

Examination I-2

Directions

Remove Examination I-2 from the manual. First, take a careful look at the examination. There should be 100 examination items. Notice that a blank line precedes each examination item number. This line is provided for you to enter the answer to the examination item. Write the answer in ink. Remember the rule about not changing your answers. Our research shows that changed answers are most often changed to an incorrect answer, and, more often than not, the answer that is chosen first is correct.

If you guess an answer, place an "X" or a check mark by your answer. This step is vitally important to gain and master knowledge. We will explain how we treat the "guessed" items later in SAEP.

Take the examination. Once you complete it, go to Appendix A and score your examination. After the examination is scored, carefully follow the directions for feedback of the missed and guessed examination items.

_____ 1. When patients become trapped or pinned within an automobile, _____ is necessary to disentangle them from the wreckage.
  A. cribbing
  B. entrapment
  C. extrication
  D. triage

_____ 2. _____ are markings on vehicles and buildings that alert emergency responders of the presence of hazardous materials.
  A. Response guides
  B. Placards
  C. Guidebook markings
  D. Alert tags
  E. Shipping papers

_____ 3. When packaging a patient for transport by aeromedical helicopter, an effective practice that improves safety is:
  A. patients should never be backboarded.
  B. first responders should not bother packaging the patient and should wait for the helicopter crew.
  C. never bandage any wounds or apply splints before the helicopter arrives.
  D. package the patient with all loose items covered or contained.
  E. All of the above.

_____ 4. When walking toward an aeromedical helicopter on the ground, never approach from:
  A. the rear.
  B. upwind.
  C. the front.
  D. the left side.
  E. the right side.

_____ **5.** For safety purposes, compressed gases, including oxygen, have been coded through a _____ that allows only the gas intended for the regulator to be used.
   A. gas-index system
   B. gas compression system
   C. supplemental oxygen system
   D. cylinder assembly system
   E. pin-indexing system

_____ **6.** The exchange of oxygen and carbon dioxide during the act of breathing is called:
   A. inspiration.
   B. expiration.
   C. transportation.
   D. respiration.

_____ **7.** The heart is made of muscle cells which require a constant supply of oxygen to contract. The moment both heartbeat and respirations stop is called:
   A. biological death.
   B. clinical death.
   C. cardiac arrest.
   D. end organ failure.

_____ **8.** When breathing stops or **is not** adequate enough, the body cells become saturated with a poison from the accumulation of:
   A. carbon monoxide.
   B. carbon dioxide.
   C. hydrogen peroxide.
   D. oxygen.

_____ **9.** All of the following are signs and symptoms which show an increase in carbon dioxide **except**:
   A. drowsiness.
   B. salivation.
   C. panting.
   D. hallucinations.

_____ **10.** The law of physics that governs respiration during the inspiration process is:
   A. as volume increases, pressure increases.
   B. as volume increases, pressure decreases.
   C. as volume decreases, pressure decreases.
   D. as pressure decreases, volume remains the same.

_____ **11.** When the diaphragm muscle contracts, the size of the chest cavity above it:
   A. doubles in size.
   B. remains the same.
   C. decreases.
   D. increases.

_____ **12.** Expiration is a/an _____ process.
  A. aerobic
  B. passive
  C. active
  D. anaerobic

_____ **13.** An open wound can be all of the following, <u>except</u>:
  A. penetrating puncture wound.
  B. avulsion.
  C. bruise.
  D. amputation.
  E. All of the above.

_____ **14.** Any full thickness burn is considered:
  A. first degree.
  B. second degree.
  C. third degree.
  D. fourth degree.

_____ **15.** Spurting blood that is bright red in color is typically _____ bleeding.
  A. venous
  B. capillary
  C. infectious
  D. arterial
  E. femoral

_____ **16.** _____ is the delivery of oxygen to the tissues and organs of the body.
  A. Blood pressure
  B. Perfusion
  C. Edema
  D. Hypotension
  E. Hypertension

_____ **17.** Which of the following signs and symptoms <u>is not</u> associated with hypoperfusion/shock?
  A. Red skin color
  B. Weak and rapid pulse
  C. Restlessness and anxiety
  D. Nausea and vomiting
  E. Decreased level of consciousness

_____ **18.** Inadequate functioning of the heart can result in _____ shock.
  A. metabolic
  B. respiratory
  C. septic
  D. hypovolemic
  E. cardiogenic

_____ **19.** Which of the following **is** **not** one of the four chambers of the heart?
    A. The inferior vena cava
    B. The right atrium
    C. The left ventricle
    D. The right ventricle
    E. The left atrium

_____ **20.** A newborn who is struggling to breathe should **always** be given:
    A. back blows.
    B. chest thrusts.
    C. oxygen.
    D. mouth-to-mouth resuscitation.

_____ **21.** During an abnormal delivery, the newborn's buttocks or both feet are presented and delivered first. This is called a/an:
    A. inverted presentation.
    B. breech birth.
    C. dorsal premier.
    D. premature birth.

_____ **22.** A baby weighing less than 5 ½ lbs. at birth or is born prior to the thirty-seventh week is considered:
    A. prolapsed.
    B. breech.
    C. stillborn.
    D. premature.

_____ **23.** The pulse rate of a pregnant woman is _____ than the average woman who **is** **not** pregnant.
    A. faster
    B. slower
    C. steadier
    D. no different

_____ **24.** The greatest danger to a pregnant mother and her unborn child during a trauma emergency is bleeding and:
    A. multiple sclerosis.
    B. breech birth.
    C. placenta abruptus.
    D. shock.

_____ **25.** If a patient requiring CPR is a child or infant, _____, then alert the EMS dispatcher (call 911).
    A. begin CPR immediately, and call for the parents
    B. begin CPR immediately, and continue for one minute
    C. wait until parents give consent, then start CPR
    D. wait until help arrives

_____ **26.** The ratio of breaths to compressions in one-rescuer CPR is:
  A. 1: 5.
  B. 2: 15.
  C. 1: 15.
  D. 2: 10.

_____ **27.** The compression rate for adult CPR is:
  A. as fast as possible.
  B. 60–80 per minute.
  C. 120 per minute.
  D. 100 per minute.

_____ **28.** Once CPR is started, you should check for signs of circulation after:
  A. 20 seconds.
  B. 15 seconds.
  C. one minute.
  D. one cycle of compressions/ventilations.

_____ **29.** On a child, the location for checking a pulse is the:
  A. brachial artery.
  B. radial artery.
  C. carotid artery.
  D. femoral artery.

_____ **30.** On an infant, the location for checking a pulse is the:
  A. brachial artery.
  B. radial artery.
  C. carotid artery.
  D. femoral artery.

_____ **31.** For a child over _____, use adult CPR techniques.
  A. 20 kilograms
  B. 16 years old
  C. 50 lbs.
  D. 8 years old

_____ **32.** The correct volume for each breath is:
  A. 15 l/kg.
  B. 400 cc.
  C. the volume that causes the chest to rise.
  D. your maximum expiratory volume.

_____ **33.** In the case of a neonate, if the heart rate is less than 60 beats per minute or between 60 and 80 beats per minute and not increasing, you should:
  A. continue to assist ventilations and begin chest compressions.
  B. support ventilations only.
  C. administer blow-by oxygen.
  D. perform chest compressions at a rate of 40 to 60 per minute.

_____ **34.** A _____ is a point where bones connect to other bones.
   A. cavity
   B. rotation point
   C. joint
   D. fontanel
   E. connection

_____ **35.** Which of the following **is** **not** a type of muscle found in the human body?
   A. Cardiac muscle
   B. Smooth muscle
   C. Proximal muscle
   D. Skeletal muscle

_____ **36.** What type of muscle can generate its own electrical impulse?
   A. Skeletal
   B. Cardiac
   C. Proximal
   D. Smooth
   E. Voluntary

_____ **37.** A system which protects the body from disease-causing organisms is known as the _____ system.
   A. endocrine
   B. urinary
   C. musculoskeletal
   D. immune

_____ **38.** The inferior portion of the sternum is known as the:
   A. intercoastal arch.
   B. xiphoid process.
   C. umbilicus.
   D. diaphragm.

_____ **39.** Which of the following **is** **not** a function performed by the skin?
   A. Protects the body from the environment
   B. Helps regulate body temperature
   C. Secretes hormones
   D. Helps prevent dehydration/regulates body fluids and chemical balance
   E. Provides sensory input such as temperature and pressure

_____ **40.** A condition in infants that causes them to have periods in which they **do** **not** breathe while sleeping is called:
   A. croup.
   B. nocturnal dyspnea.
   C. apnea.
   D. epiglottis.

_____ **41.** A sudden, unexplained death during sleep of an apparently healthy baby in his or her first year of life is called:
A. Sudden Infant Death Syndrome (SIDS).
B. Proximal Nocturnal Dyspnea.
C. Sudden Infant Apnea Syndrome.
D. Infantile Febrile Seizure Disorder.

_____ **42.** A child or infant who has suffered from an excessive loss of body fluid through vomiting and/or diarrhea is:
A. dehydrated.
B. hypothermic.
C. seizing.
D. in respiratory distress.

_____ **43.** Specified treatment plans and actions that emergency medical providers use in caring for certain types of emergencies are:
A. patient plans.
B. medical suggestions.
C. prescriptions.
D. treatment maps.
E. protocols.

_____ **44.** The **most** **advanced** level of emergency medical care training as defined by the United States Department of transportation (DOT) is the:
A. first responder.
B. emergency medical technician-basic (EMT-B).
C. emergency medical technician-intermediate (EMT-I).
D. emergency medical technician-enhanced (EMT-E).
E. emergency medical technician-paramedic (EMT-P).

_____ **45.** A first responder treating a patient based on local protocols is an example of _____ medical control.
A. indirect (off-line)
B. inherent
C. direct (online)
D. intermediate

_____ **46.** What is the **next** step to follow once an emergency occurs and it is recognized?
A. Activate the AED
B. Start CPR
C. Perform primary survey
D. Activate the EMS system

_____ **47.** A member of the EMS system who is trained to provide first care to a patient and assist EMTs at an emergency scene is called a:
A. bystander.
B. first responder.
C. community service aide.
D. medical director.

_____ **48.** Which of the following **is not** an element of negligence?
   A. Duty
   B. Breach of duty
   C. Abandonment
   D. Causation of injury
   E. Damages

_____ **49.** A first responder who treats a patient without consent may be charged with:
   A. abandonment.
   B. causation of injury.
   C. breach of jury.
   D. assault, battery, or false imprisonment.
   E. emancipation.

_____ **50.** _____ are directions a person describes for family members and
   caregivers in advance of a life-threatening situation or condition.
   A. Advance directives
   B. Resuscitation orders
   C. Confidentiality agreements
   D. Liability instructions
   E. Consent directives

_____ **51.** A/An _____ directs that resuscitative efforts **not** be initiated in the case of
   cardiac or respiratory arrest if it is determined that resuscitation would
   prolong suffering.
   A. pre-consent agreement
   B. Do Not Resuscitate (DNR) order
   C. express consent override
   D. causation clause
   E. medical care request

_____ **52.** When no parent or legal guardian is present and a child has a life- or limb-
   threatening emergency, what type of consent do first responders have to treat
   the child?
   A. Implied consent
   B. Express consent
   C. Emancipated consent
   D. Competent consent
   E. Pediatric consent

_____ **53.** What types of activities can the first responder do to improve lifting and
   moving skills and abilities?
   A. Improve personal fitness.
   B. Perform cardiovascular exercise.
   C. Work as a team with other first responders.
   D. All of the above.

_____ **54.** Which of the following **best** describes the patient movement situation for a patient in immediate danger?
A. Nonurgent move
B. Emergency move
C. Position of comfort
D. Stabilization move

_____ **55.** When lifting a patient or object you must estimate the patient's _____ first.
A. age
B. height
C. weight
D. girth

_____ **56.** The greatest danger to a patient during an emergency move is the possibility of:
A. making a spinal cord injury worse.
B. being dropped by the rescuer.
C. cross contamination.
D. resumption of bleeding.

_____ **57.** The line that runs down the center of the body from the top of the head and along the spine is called:
A. transverse segment.
B. the long axis of the body.
C. inferior digitalis.
D. Angle of Louis.

_____ **58.** The _____ phase is the state following a seizure in which the patient may be sleepy, confused, or hostile.
A. acute
B. febrile
C. grand mal
D. status epilepticus
E. postictal

_____ **59.** Hypoglycemia refers to:
A. low blood sugar.
B. pale moist skin.
C. headache.
D. shallow breathing.

_____ **60.** Which of the following objects can be used in an emergency between the teeth of a convulsing patient?
A. Wallet
B. Oropharyngeal airway
C. Bite stick
D. Nothing should be placed in the patient's mouth.

_____ **61.** Which of the following **is** **not** considered appropriate emergency care for a suspected stroke patient?
A. Administer two baby aspirins
B. Ensure an open airway
C. Treat for shock
D. Place the patient into the recovery position

_____ **62.** <u>Scenario</u>: While watching television, a wife notices her husband suddenly becomes unable to speak. He had been complaining of a headache earlier in the evening. You suspect the husband has suffered:
A. a heart attack.
B. gastritis.
C. a stroke.
D. pancreatitis.

_____ **63.** Signs and symptoms of respiratory distress include all of the following **except**:
A. blue coloration.
B. miosis.
C. altered mental status.
D. noisy respirations.

_____ **64.** A/An _____ is a system for managing and controlling the resources on an emergency scene so that the response and actions are organized and efficient.
A. triage system/AVPU system
B. mass casualty system
C. placarding system
D. incident management system/incident command system

_____ **65.** The technique of applying a/an _____ is used to immobilize shoulder and arm injuries.
A. air splint
B. vacuum splint
C. splint and spine board
D. sling and swathe

_____ **66.** A process of immobilizing and stabilizing painful, swollen, deformed extremities is known as:
A. setting.
B. splinting.
C. pinning.
D. alleviating.

_____ **67.** The three main signs and symptoms in an extremity fracture include deformity, pain, and:
A. full range of motion.
B. brisk capillary refill.
C. symmetry.
D. swelling.

_____ **68.** Which **is** **not** one of the forces that cause musculoskeletal injuries?
  A. Anaerobic force
  B. Direct force
  C. Twisting force
  D. Indirect forc

_____ **69.** The main reason to straighten closed deformed injuries (if EMS system allows first responders to do so) is:
  A. to control bleeding.
  B. ease of transport.
  C. to improve blood flow.
  D. to provide pain relief.

_____ **70.** The musculoskeletal system has four major functions which include support, protection, producing blood cells, and:
  A. immunity.
  B. glucose production.
  C. movement.
  D. sensory transmission.

_____ **71.** Parts of the body that enable us to move and function, such as muscles, joints, bones, tendons, and ligaments make up the:
  A. musculoskeletal system.
  B. exoskeleton system.
  C. circulatory system.
  D. lymphatic system.

_____ **72.** Sporadic noises coming from a patient's airway without any chest movement is called:
  A. agonal respirations.
  B. snoring respirations.
  C. spastic respirations.
  D. apnea.

_____ **73.** The normal return/refill of capillaries after blood has been forced out by fingertip pressure applied to a patient's nail bed (is):
  A. 5 seconds or less.
  B. varies with age.
  C. 2 seconds or less.
  D. 10 seconds.

_____ **74.** Vital signs consist of pulse, pupils, relative skin color, condition, temperature, and:
  A. physical examination.
  B. respirations.
  C. secondary survey.
  D. blood alcohol level.

_____ **75.** All of the following represent significant mechanisms of injury **except**:
  A. falls greater than 15 feet.
  B. ejection from a vehicle.
  C. flail chest.
  D. vehicle-pedestrian collision.

_____ **76.** A first responder's **best** source of information is from:
  A. the vial of life.
  B. family members and bystanders.
  C. medical records.
  D. a responsive and alert patient.

_____ **77.** Which of the following is/are reasons to inquire about the patient's last oral intake?
  A. A full stomach slows medical absorption.
  B. Possible diabetic emergency
  C. Patient must fast prior to blood tests.
  D. Hospitals may not feed a patient for quite some time.

_____ **78.** The term DCAP-BTLS includes all of the following **except**:
  A. contusions.
  B. tenderness.
  C. avulsions.
  D. swelling.

_____ **79.** The absence of a radial pulse when there is a carotid pulse indicates possible:
  A. hypertension.
  B. pulsus parodixus.
  C. tissue necrosis.
  D. shock.

_____ **80.** The rapid trauma assessment is a head-to-toe physical exam that should take:
  A. place in back of the rescue.
  B. no more than one minute.
  C. no more than two to three minutes.
  D. at least four minutes.

_____ **81.** What is the acronym used to determine how the patient responds and to evaluate the level of consciousness?
  A. PERL
  B. SAMPLE
  C. AVPU
  D. OPQRST

_____ **82.** For the ongoing assessment, critical patients should be reassessed every _____ minute(s) and stable patients every _____ minutes.
  A. 1; 5
  B. 5; 7
  C. 5; 15
  D. 10; 15
  E. 10; 20

_____ **83.** The important components to gather when interviewing a patient are the signs and symptoms, _____, medications, past medical history, last oral intake, and the events preceding the onset of complaint.
  A. abdominal problems
  B. allergies
  C. alertness
  D. airway problems

_____ **84.** Hypotension is defined as a systolic blood pressure less than _____ mm Hg.
  A. 40
  B. 68
  C. 90
  D. 100
  E. 120

_____ **85.** Which of the following techniques can be used to measure a patient's response to painful stimuli?
  A. Sternal rub
  B. Pinching the ear lobe
  C. Pinching the skin on an upper extremity
  D. All of the above.

_____ **86.** A rapid heart rate that is greater than 100 beats per minute is called:
  A. bradycardia.
  B. asystole.
  C. ventricular fibrillation.
  D. atrial fibrillation.
  E. tachycardia.

_____ **87.** What is the range of normal respiratory rates for adult patients?
  A. 6–8
  B. 12–20
  C. 15–40
  D. 20–40
  E. 40–60

_____ **88.** Critical incident stress debriefing (CISD) usually begins with a _____ that occurs a few hours after the critical incident and is short and informal.
  A. counseling session
  B. debriefing
  C. critique
  D. defusing
  E. team meeting

_____ **89.** Which of the following **is not** an element of the Critical Incident Stress Management system?
   A. Leadership coaching
   B. Disaster support services
   C. On-scene support
   D. Community outreach programs
   E. Support for spouses and families

_____ **90.** In the CISD process, a structured meeting called a _____ usually occurs within 24 to 72 hours after a critical incident.
   A. counseling session
   B. debriefing
   C. critique
   D. defusing
   E. team meeting

_____ **91.** A type of incident that may cause a first responder to experience critical incident stress is one that involves:
   A. a multiple casualty incident or disaster.
   B. children.
   C. death or injury of a co-worker.
   D. All of the above.

_____ **92.** All of the following are means of safeguarding your physical and emotional well-being **except**:
   A. ensuring scene safety.
   B. an annual psychological review.
   C. using universal precautions/including PPE.
   D. learning about stressors.

_____ **93.** More healthcare workers die each year from _____ or its complications than from any other infectious disease.
   A. Human Immunodeficiency Virus (HIV)
   B. hepatitis B (HBV)
   C. Acquired Immune Deficiency Syndrome (AIDS)
   D. hepatitis C (HCV)

_____ **94.** Trying to understand the feelings of the patient or family member is an example of:
   A. empathy.
   B. apathy.
   C. sympathy.
   D. tolerance.

_____ **95.** _____ is/are a form of infection control based on the presumption that all body fluids are infectious.
   A. Body substance isolation
   B. Disease protocols
   C. Universal protocols
   D. Impermeable barriers

_____ **96.** Difficulty sleeping, loss of appetite, and inability to concentrate are all warning signs of:
A. type A personality.
B. job burn-out.
C. diabetes.
D. stress.

_____ **97.** All of the following are examples of infection control barriers **except**:
A. pocket face mask with one way valve.
B. eye shields.
C. nonrebreathing mask.
D. latex or vinyl gloves.

_____ **98.** _____ are agents produced by the body to combat specific microorganisms.
A. Pathogens
B. Innoculations
C. Carriers
D. Antibodies

_____ **99.** Needles used for intravenous access or injections **must** be disposed of in a:
A. regular waste container or trash receptacle.
B. biohazardous bag (red bag).
C. dumpster.
D. sharps container (hard plastic container).

_____**100.** What type of disease transmission is caused by touching a substance that contains an infectious agent?
A. Direct contact
B. Airborne transmission
C. Carrier-based
D. Vector-borne transmission

—————— **Helpful Hint** ——————
Try to determine why you selected the wrong answer. Usually something influenced your selection. Focus on the difference between your wrong answer and the correct answer. Carefully read and study the entire paragraph containing the correct answer. Highlight the answer just as you did for Examination I-1.

Did you score higher than 80 percent on Examination I-2? Circle Yes or No in ink. (**We will return to your answer to this question later in SAEP.**)

Now that you have finished the Feedback Step for Examination I-2, it is time to repeat the process by taking another comprehensive examination of the *DOT, First Responder National Standard Curriculum.*

Examination I-3, Confirming What You Mastered

During Examination I-3, progress will be made in reinforcing what you have learned and improving your examination-taking skills. This examination contains approximately 60 percent of the examination items you have already answered and several new examination items. Follow the steps carefully to realize the best return on effort.

Step 1—Take Examination I-3. When you have completed Examination I-3, go to Appendix A and compare your answers with the correct answers.

Step 2—Score Examination I-3. How many examination items did you miss? Write the number of missed examination items in the blank in ink _____. Enter the number of examination items you guessed in this blank _____. Enter these numbers in the designated locations on your Personal Progress Plotter.

Step 3—During the feedback step, research the correct answer using the Appendix A information for Examination I-3. Highlight the correct answer during your research of the reference materials. Read the entire paragraph containing the correct answer.

Examination I-3

Directions

Remove Examination I-3 from the manual. First, take a careful look at the examination. There should be 150 examination items. Notice that a blank line precedes each examination item number. This line is provided for you to enter the answer to the examination item. Write the answer in ink. Remember the rule about not changing your answers. Our research shows that changed answers are most often changed to an incorrect answer, and, more often than not, the answer that is chosen first is correct.

If you guess an answer, place an "X" or a check mark by your answer. This step is vitally important to gain and master knowledge. We will explain how we treat the "guessed" items later in SAEP.

Take the examination. Once you complete it, go to Appendix A and score your examination. Once the examination is scored, carefully follow the directions for feedback of the missed and guessed examination items.

_____ **1.** All of the following tools can be used to help unlock a vehicle door **except** a:
- **A.** slim-jim.
- **B.** screwdriver.
- **C.** wire hook.
- **D.** K Tool.

_____ **2.** _____ are markings on vehicles and buildings that alert emergency responders of the presence of hazardous materials.
- **A.** Response guides
- **B.** Placards
- **C.** Guidebook markings
- **D.** Alert tags
- **E.** Shipping papers

_____ **3.** A helicopter landing zone should be _____ during nighttime hours.
- **A.** 60' X 75'
- **B.** 75' X 75'
- **C.** 85' X 90'
- **D.** 100' X 100'

_____ **4.** The _____ is a tubular structure that begins below the vocal cords and extends into the chest and carries air into and out of the lungs.
- **A.** bronchi
- **B.** alveoli
- **C.** trachea
- **D.** epiglottis
- **E.** bronchioles

_____ **5.** The **best** method of opening the airway in patients who have suffered or potentially suffered a traumatic injury is:
- **A.** the head tilt–chin lift method.
- **B.** the jaw thrust.
- **C.** the nasopharyngeal method.
- **D.** All of the above methods.

_____ **6.** Suctioning should be performed for no longer than _____ seconds in adult patients.
   A. 5
   B. 10
   C. 15
   D. 20
   E. 25

_____ **7.** The heart is made of muscle cells which require a constant supply of oxygen to contract. The moment both heartbeat and respirations stop is called:
   A. biological death.
   B. clinical death.
   C. cardiac arrest.
   D. end organ failure.

_____ **8.** The law of physics that governs respiration during the inspiration process is:
   A. as volume increases, pressure increases.
   B. as volume increases, pressure decreases.
   C. as volume decreases, pressure decreases.
   D. as pressure decreases, volume remains the same.

_____ **9.** The flap of tissue that is located above the larynx whose purpose is to close off the airway when a person swallows is called the:
   A. epidermis.
   B. xyphoid process.
   C. epiglottis.
   D. pharynx.

_____ **10.** All of the following are signs of a complete airway obstruction **except**:
   A. a conscious patient will try to speak or cough and will be unable to do so.
   B. the patient will often grasp their neck and open their mouth widely.
   C. an unconscious patient will not have any of the typical chest movements or other signs of good air exchange.
   D. whistling heard upon inspiration.

_____ **11.** All of the following are common problems associated with the mouth-to-barrier resuscitation technique **except** failure to:
   A. clear airway of obstructions.
   B. pinch the nose completely closed.
   C. form a tight seal over the patient's mouth.
   D. observe adequate chest rise.

_____ **12.** Small sacs inside the lungs where oxygen and carbon dioxide are exchanged are:
   A. bladders.
   B. bronchioles.
   C. tracheas.
   D. oropharynx.
   E. alveoli.

_____ **13.** The _____ is the passageway connecting the upper airway to the lungs.
  A. alveoli
  B. nasopharynx
  C. oropharynx
  D. trachea

_____ **14.** _____ is a high pitched respiratory sound when breathing caused by narrowing of the airway due to obstruction.
  A. Fontanel
  B. Cervix
  C. Grunting
  D. Stridor
  E. Coughing

_____ **15.** To provide proper circulatory function, a typical adult must maintain a volume of _____ liters of blood.
  A. 5–6
  B. 7–8
  C. 3–4
  D. 9–10

_____ **16.** You should **not** use elevation in combination with direct pressure when dealing with:
  A. the amputation of an extremity.
  B. a possible extremity fracture.
  C. muscle lesions.
  D. a pelvic fracture.

_____ **17.** There are 22 major pressure point sites used to control bleeding (11 sites on each side of the body). Which two sites are commonly part of first responder training?
  A. Carotid
  B. Carpel pedal
  C. Brachial and femoral
  D. Radial

_____ **18.** An internal injury causing blood vessels and organs to be crushed or ruptured by a severe blow to the body, but with no cuts to the skin is a type of:
  A. systemic laceration.
  B. avulsion.
  C. penetrating trauma.
  D. blunt trauma.

_____ **19.** Spurting blood that is bright red in color is typically _____ bleeding.
  A. venous
  B. capillary
  C. infectious
  D. arterial
  E. femoral

_____ **20.** Which of the following **is not** one of the four chambers of the heart?
  A. The inferior vena cava
  B. The right atrium
  C. The left ventricle
  D. The right ventricle
  E. The left atrium

_____ **21.** If bleeding saturates the original bandage placed on the injury site, the first responder should:
  A. remove the original bandage and replace it with a new bandage.
  B. remove the original bandage and replace it with a larger bandage.
  C. place a heat pack over the original bandage site.
  D. apply another layer of sterile dressing or bandaging over the original bandage.
  E. discontinue trying to bandage the wound.

_____ **22.** Which of the following are burns to the outer layer of skin only?
  A. Partial thickness burns
  B. Superficial burns
  C. Full thickness burns
  D. Electrical burns

_____ **23.** A/An _____ dressing should be applied to penetrating wounds of the chest.
  A. pressure
  B. occlusive
  C. full thickness
  D. thermal
  E. thorax

_____ **24.** A/An _____ occurs when capillaries under the skin bleed causing blood to pool in the soft tissues under the skin.
  A. contusion
  B. avulsion
  C. abrasion
  D. laceration
  E. amputation

_____ **25.** Labor pains normally come at regular intervals and last for about:
  A. 2 to 3 minutes.
  B. 30 seconds to 1 minute.
  C. 30 minutes to 1 hour.
  D. 3 to 4 minutes.

_____ **26.** Consider a birth delivery to be normal if:
  A. it lasts only five minutes.
  B. the baby's head appears first.
  C. the feet present first.
  D. the shoulders appear first.

_____ **27.** The greatest danger to a pregnant mother and her unborn child during a trauma emergency is bleeding and:
    A. multiple sclerosis.
    B. breech birth.
    C. placenta abruptus.
    D. shock.

_____ **28.** The _____ is a hollow muscular organ located in the female pelvic cavity that serves as the implantation site for the fertilized egg.
    A. cervix
    B. ovary
    C. uterus
    D. vagina

_____ **29.** The _____ fluid surrounds the fetus providing a cushion of protection.
    A. vaginal
    B. cervix
    C. placental
    D. amniotic

_____ **30.** What occurs during the second stage of labor?
    A. The baby is delivered.
    B. The baby rotates within the uterus.
    C. The cervix dilates.
    D. The placenta is delivered.
    E. Bloody show is expelled.

_____ **31.** Which of the following statements about AEDs is **false**?
    A. AEDs require the user to interpret the cardiac rhythm.
    B. AEDs should be inspected regularly.
    C. First responders should check the batteries on the AED unit per the manufacturer's recommendations.
    D. AED pouches often carry extra supplies like razors and gauze.
    E. Some AEDs have a screen that displays the heart rhythm.

_____ **32.** In which of the following situations can an AED be used?
    A. A conscious patient experiencing trouble breathing
    B. A patient in cardiac arrest
    C. An unconscious child who has a pulse
    D. A conscious adult having chest pain
    E. All of the above.

_____ **33.** Which of the statements about using an AED is **true**?
    A. While the AED is analyzing the patient's rhythm, it is acceptable to be touching the patient or continue performing CPR.
    B. The AED will ask the user to interpret the heart rhythm.
    C. CPR must be stopped for the entire cycle of analysis for the AED to accurately assess the patient's heart rhythm.
    D. Local protocols are not important to the first responder regarding the use of AEDs.
    E. First responders should immediately attach an AED to every patient.

_____ **34.** If a patient in cardiac arrest is found with a bulge in the chest thought to be an artificial pacemaker, the first responder should:

   A. place the AED electrode directly on top of the bulge in the chest.

   B. place the AED electrode to the left of the bulge and several inches lower (toward the feet).

   C. place both AED electrodes on the lower left ribcage area.

   D. discontinue use of the AED.

   E. place the AED electrode on the shoulder above the bulge.

_____ **35.** _____ are the pads in contact with a patient's skin that allow electrical impulses to be read by a heart monitor, and allow the delivery of an electrical defibrillation if necessary.

   A. Dysrhythmias

   B. Electrodes

   C. Electrocardiograms

   D. Contraindications

   E. Medication patches

_____ **36.** The ratio of breaths to compressions in one rescuer CPR is:

   A. 1:5.

   B. 2:15.

   C. 1:15.

   D. 2:10.

_____ **37.** The compression rate for adult CPR is:

   A. as fast as possible.

   B. 60–80 per minute.

   C. 120 per minute.

   D. 100 per minute.

_____ **38.** Once CPR is started, you should check for signs of circulation after:

   A. 20 seconds.

   B. 15 seconds.

   C. one minute.

   D. one cycle of compressions/ventilations.

_____ **39.** On a child, the location for checking a pulse is the:

   A. brachial artery.

   B. radial artery.

   C. carotid artery.

   D. femoral artery.

_____ **40.** On an infant, the location for checking a pulse is the:

   A. brachial artery.

   B. radial artery.

   C. carotid artery.

   D. femoral artery.

_____ **41.** For a child over _____, use adult CPR techniques.
  A. 20 kilograms
  B. 16 years old
  C. 50 lbs.
  D. 8 years old

_____ **42.** In a diving accident, suspect neck injury and use the _____ to open the airway.
  A. head tilt–chin lift
  B. jaw thrust maneuver
  C. modified head tilt–chin lift
  D. Sellick's maneuver

_____ **43.** Which of the following heart rhythms can be corrected with defibrillation?
  A. Regular sinus rhythm
  B. Asystole
  C. Ventricular fibrillation
  D. Sinus bradycardia

_____ **44.** During two-rescuer CPR, the **best** time to check for return of respirations and pulses is:
  A. after one minute or four cycles.
  B. after 5 minutes of CPR.
  C. in between cycles of compressions and ventilations.
  D. whenever conveniently done.

_____ **45.** All of the following are reasons why two-rescuer CPR, when performed correctly, is more efficient than one-rescuer CPR **except**:
  A. rescuer fatigue is reduced.
  B. more personnel are required.
  C. patient receives more oxygen.
  D. compression rate allows for better filling of the heart.

_____ **46.** During two-rescuer CPR, breathing and carotid pulse should be checked after the _____ minute, and then every _____ minutes.
  A. fifth, two
  B. fifth, ten
  C. third, three
  D. first, few

_____ **47.** While changing positions during two-rescuer CPR, the first responder now ventilating checks for a carotid pulse and states, "No Pulse, _____"
  A. call for back-up.
  B. continue CPR.
  C. what do I do next?
  D. administer a precordial thump.

_____ **48.** The front of the body is referred to as:
   A. posterior.
   B. medial.
   C. proximal.
   D. anterior.
   E. distal.

_____ **49.** The <u>lowest</u> point on the sternum, which is used as a landmark for locating proper hand position during CPR, is the:
   A. coccyx.
   B. fontanel.
   C. xiphoid process.
   D. thorax.
   E. diaphragm.

_____ **50.** The muscle that separates the thoracic and abdominal cavities is the:
   A. pectorals.
   B. xiphoid process.
   C. trapezius.
   D. thorax.
   E. diaphragm.

_____ **51.** The three main components of the circulatory system are the _____, the blood vessels, and the blood.
   A. aorta
   B. stomach
   C. heart
   D. coronary arteries
   E. pancreas

_____ **52.** The inferior portion of the sternum is known as the:
   A. intercostal arch.
   B. xiphoid process.
   C. umbilicus.
   D. diaphragm.

_____ **53.** Which of the following organs **is** **not** found in the digestive system?
   A. Gall bladder
   B. Stomach
   C. Liver
   D. Small intestine
   E. Uterus

_____ **54.** Which of the following organs is found in a male human's reproductive system?
   A. Cervix
   B. Uterus
   C. Prostate gland
   D. Ovaries
   E. Fallopian tubes

_____ **55.** The exchange of air to bring in oxygen and expel carbon dioxide is known as the _____ system.
- **A.** circulatory
- **B.** digestive
- **C.** nervous
- **D.** respiratory

_____ **56.** To perform a _____ the first responder must be familiar with the normal anatomy of the human body.
- **A.** Heimlich maneuver
- **B.** patient extrication
- **C.** patient assessment
- **D.** patient transfer

_____ **57.** The anatomical position refers to:
- **A.** standing erect, facing the observer, arms down at the sides, with palms facing forward.
- **B.** standing erect, facing the observer, arms over the head, with palms facing forward.
- **C.** lying on the left side, arms down at the sides, with palms facing forward.
- **D.** standing erect, facing the observer, arms down at the sides, with palms facing backward.

_____ **58.** What is referred to as toward the feet?
- **A.** Superior
- **B.** Anterior
- **C.** Posterior
- **D.** Inferior

_____ **59.** All of the following help to make up the upper and lower extremities **except** the:
- **A.** knee.
- **B.** sternum.
- **C.** forearm.
- **D.** wrist.
- **E.** ankle.

_____ **60.** At times, a first responder will be unable to determine the age of an infant or child; therefore, an estimate of age can be determined based on all of the following **except**:
- **A.** physical size.
- **B.** level of consciousness.
- **C.** emotional responses.
- **D.** interaction with the first responder.
- **E.** language skills.

61. If a suspected hip or pelvis injury has occurred in a child, you should do all of the following **except**:
  A. monitor vital signs for shock.
  B. rock the hips to check for instability.
  C. check for bleeding or bloody discharge from the genital area.
  D. arrange for transport as soon as possible.

62. A sudden, unexplained death during sleep of an apparently healthy baby in his or her first year of life is called:
  A. Sudden Infant Death Syndrome (SIDS).
  B. Proximal Nocturnal Dyspnea.
  C. Sudden Infant Apnea Syndrome.
  D. Infantile Febrile Seizure Disorder.

63. _____ is defined as giving insufficient attention or respect to someone who has a claim to that attention.
  A. Child abuse
  B. Child abandonment
  C. Child neglect
  D. Shaken baby syndrome
  E. Sudden infant death syndrome

64. Which of the following statements is **false** regarding pediatric anatomy and physiology?
  A. Infants and children have proportionally larger heads than adults.
  B. There are really no significant differences between adults and pediatric patients with regard to anatomy and physiology.
  C. The trachea in an infant is small and fragile and more easily obstructed.
  D. Infants have fontanels on the skull.
  E. A jaw thrust airway opening maneuver is used when infants or children have a traumatic injury.

65. The extent of medical procedures a first responder is authorized to perform is called the:
  A. medical release.
  B. scope of practice/care.
  C. duty to act.
  D. physician relationship.
  E. skill set.

66. _____ is a formal relationship between the emergency medical service providers and the physician responsible for out-of-hospital emergency medical care.
  A. Medical monitoring
  B. Health care tracking
  C. Provider monitoring
  D. Medical oversight
  E. Physician tracking

_____ **67.** What kind of medical control occurs when no direct contact is made with a physician in the course of treating a patient?

  A. Indirect (off-line) medical control
  B. Inherent medical control
  C. Direct (online) medical control
  D. Intermediate medical control
  E. Online medical control

_____ **68.** A first responder treating a patient based on local protocols is an example of _____ medical control.

  A. indirect (off-line)
  B. inherent
  C. direct (online)
  D. intermediate

_____ **69.** A member of the EMS system who is trained to provide first care to a patient and assist EMTs at an emergency scene is called a:

  A. bystander.
  B. first responder.
  C. community service aide.
  D. medical director.

_____ **70.** In an enhanced 911 system, the dispatcher is trained to help and instruct bystanders in all of the following **except**:

  A. protecting the patient.
  B. receiving caller information.
  C. reading the patient's Miranda Rights.
  D. providing pre-arrival care instructions.

_____ **71.** Personal protection from possible contact with infectious agents may require the use of all of the following **except**:

  A. gowns or aprons.
  B. protective eyewear (goggles or face shields).
  C. approved latex or vinyl gloves.
  D. radiation badges.

_____ **72.** The **number** **one** concern of any first responder should be:

  A. the safety of the patient.
  B. safe driving.
  C. the safety of bystanders.
  D. personal safety.
  E. the safety of other team members.

_____ **73.** A patient who is awake and alert and who verbalizes her consent for the first responder to provide care has given:

  A. implied consent.
  B. express consent.
  C. emancipated consent.
  D. competent consent.
  E. inherent consent.

_____ **74.** What term describes the ability of a patient to understand questions, act responsibly, and comprehend the implications of decisions?
A. Consent
B. Emancipation
C. Liability
D. Competence
E. Causation

_____ **75.** _____ is a deviation from the accepted standard of care resulting in further injury to a patient.
A. Abandonment
B. Breaching
C. Causation
D. Liability
E. Negligence

_____ **76.** The level of care that is expected as based on the provider's training and experience within the limitations imposed by an emergency situation is called:
A. level of accountability.
B. treatment modality.
C. medical control.
D. standard of care.

_____ **77.** When a minor is involved in an accident, and the parents/guardians **are not** on the scene and cannot be reached quickly, the minor can be treated under the law of:
A. minor's consent.
B. implied consent.
C. informed consent.
D. advance directives.

_____ **78.** EMS personnel can be alerted to a patient's medical condition such as allergies, diabetes, or epilepsy by:
A. advance directives.
B. medical identification devices.
C. pre-consent agreements.
D. All of the above.

_____ **79.** When lifting an object or patient, keep the weight being lifted:
A. as close to the body as possible.
B. as far away from the body as possible.
C. to the left side of the body.
D. to the right side of the body.

_____ **80.** Which of the following **is** a lifting and moving device used in emergency medical services?
A. Wheeled stretcher
B. Stair chair
C. Scoop (or orthopedic) stretcher
D. Backboard
E. All of the above.

_____ **81.** The term for the position a patient assumes to compensate for pain and discomfort is:
   A. position of comfort.
   B. recovery positioning.
   C. urgent positioning.
   D. indicated position.
   E. position of patient care.

_____ **82.** Which of the following **best** describes the patient movement situation for a patient in immediate danger?
   A. Nonurgent move
   B. Emergency move
   C. Position of comfort
   D. Stabilization move

_____ **83.** When lifting a patient or object you must estimate the patient's _____ first.
   A. age
   B. height
   C. weight
   D. girth

_____ **84.** The greatest danger to a patient during an emergency move is the possibility of:
   A. making a spinal cord injury worse.
   B. being dropped by the rescuer.
   C. cross contamination.
   D. resumption of bleeding.

_____ **85.** The line that runs down the center of the body from the top of the head and along the spine is called:
   A. transverse segment.
   B. the long axis of the body.
   C. inferior digitalis.
   D. Angle of Louis.

_____ **86.** All of the following rapid move techniques can be used in a drag **except**:
   A. dragged by the clothes.
   B. dragged by the shoulders/armpits.
   C. dragged by the legs.
   D. dragged on a blanket.

_____ **87.** On which side is the patient placed when placed in the recovery position?
   A. Left
   B. Right
   C. Supine
   D. Prone

_____ **88.** When packaging a patient on a backboard, you must also stabilize the head and neck first by using the correct type and size of _____ on the patient.
   A. oral airway
   B. cervical collar
   C. Kendrick extrication device
   D. nasopharyngeal airway

_____ **89.** _____ is a condition where the body is exposed to a cold environment and is unable to compensate for the heat loss, resulting in an abnormally low core temperature.
   A. Heat exhaustion
   B. Hypothermia
   C. Heatstroke
   D. Hyperthermia
   E. Frostbite

_____ **90.** Which of the following **is not** a potential sign or symptom of a local cold emergency?
   A. Bright red skin color
   B. Loss of feeling or sensation in the affected area
   C. Swelling
   D. Blisters
   E. Pain or numbness in the affected area

_____ **91.** Which of the following statements is **false** regarding the treatment of a patient with hypothermia and/or a local cold emergency?
   A. Attempt to break any blisters present.
   B. Refrain from rubbing or massaging injury or area involved.
   C. Do not apply heat to deep cold injuries.
   D. Refrain from allowing a patient to walk on an affected extremity.
   E. Handle patients very gently.

_____ **92.** Which of the following is the life-threatening third stage of heat exposure where body systems begin to shut down?
   A. Heat seizures
   B. Heat cramps
   C. Heatstroke
   D. Heat exhaustion
   E. Hypothermia

_____ **93.** Which of the following **is not** considered appropriate emergency care for a suspected stroke patient?
   A. Administer two baby aspirins
   B. Ensure an open airway
   C. Treat for shock
   D. Place the patient into the recovery position

_____ **94.** <u>Scenario</u>: While watching television, a wife notices her husband suddenly becomes unable to speak. He had been complaining of a headache earlier in the evening. You suspect the husband has suffered:
    A. a heart attack.
    B. gastritis.
    C. a stroke.
    D. pancreatitis.

_____ **95.** Shortness of breath, barrel chest, cyanosis, and a desire to sit up at all times are all symptoms of:
    A. Chronic Obstructive Pulmonary Disease (COPD).
    B. hypertension.
    C. carbon monoxide poisoning.
    D. cardiac asthma.

_____ **96.** _____ is a system used to prioritize patients based on severity of injury and survivability.
    A. MCI management
    B. Incident Management System (IMS)
    C. Placards
    D. Triage
    E. Accountability

_____ **97.** A/An _____ is a system for managing and controlling the resources on an emergency scene so that the response and actions are organized and efficient.
    A. triage system/AVPU system
    B. mass casualty system
    C. placarding system
    D. incident management system/incident command system

_____ **98.** Injuries to the _____ are often associated with head injuries.
    A. trachea
    B. spine/neck
    C. orbit
    D. maxilla

_____ **99.** All of the following are signs and symptoms of a brain injury <u>except</u>:
    A. bleeding or fluid from the ears.
    B. loss of consciousness.
    C. pupils that are unequal, slow or non-reactive to light.
    D. chest pain.

_____ **100.** An injury that causes blood vessels to rupture in the brain is called a/an:
    A. avulsion.
    B. concussion.
    C. laceration.
    D. contusion.

_____ **101.** When dealing with suspected extremity dislocation, it is important to remember to:
  A. splint in the position found.
  B. apply manual traction.
  C. attempt to reduce it in the field.
  D. do all of the above.

_____ **102.** Which **is** **not** one of the forces that cause musculoskeletal injuries?
  A. Anaerobic force
  B. Direct force
  C. Twisting force
  D. Indirect force

_____ **103.** The main reason to straighten closed deformed injuries (if EMS system allows first responders to do so) is:
  A. to control bleeding.
  B. ease of transport.
  C. to improve blood flow.
  D. to provide pain relief.

_____ **104.** A/An _____ is a break in a bone.
  A. avulsion
  B. fracture
  C. abrasion
  D. laceration
  E. sprain

_____ **105.** Which of the following is a potential complication of spinal injury?
  A. Difficult or inadequate breathing
  B. Paralysis
  C. Diminished sensation in extremities
  D. All of the above.

_____ **106.** Which of the following **is** **not** a section of the spinal column?
  A. Thoracic
  B. Lumbar
  C. Cervical
  D. Sacrum
  E. Pelvic

_____ **107.** A force(s) that may have caused injury is called:
  A. trauma protocol.
  B. nature of illness.
  C. mechanism of injury.
  D. gravitational prolapse.

_____108. Which of the following is/are reasons to inquire about the patient's last oral intake?
  A. A full stomach slows medical absorption.
  B. Possible diabetic emergency
  C. Patient must fast prior to blood tests.
  D. Hospitals may not feed a patient for quite some time.

_____109. For the ongoing assessment, critical patients should be reassessed every _____ minute(s) and stable patients every _____ minutes.
  A. 1; 5
  B. 5; 7
  C. 5; 15
  D. 10; 15
  E. 10; 20

_____110. A rapid heart rate that is greater than 100 beats per minute is called:
  A. bradycardia.
  B. asystole.
  C. ventricular fibrillation.
  D. atrial fibrillation.
  E. tachycardia.

_____111. Which of the following **should** **not** be considered a symptom when conducting the initial and focused assessments?
  A. Shortness of breath
  B. Abdominal tenderness or rigidity
  C. Burning sensations
  D. Dizziness/feeling faint

_____112. When performing a detailed physical exam, first responders will inspect and palpate for DOTS, which stands for deformities, open injuries, tenderness, and:
  A. symptoms.
  B. systole.
  C. severity.
  D. swelling.
  E. signs.

_____113. Which of the following conditions **is** **not** considered a priority finding in the patient assessment?
  A. Altered mental status
  B. Difficult breathing
  C. Painful, deformed swollen wrist
  D. Signs and symptoms of hypotension or shock
  E. Chest pain

_____114. Where is the **best** place to check a pulse on an infant patient?
  A. Radial artery
  B. Femoral artery
  C. Carotid artery
  D. Aorta
  E. Brachial artery

_____ **115.** Any open wounds to the chest need to be covered immediately with a/an:
  A. occlusive dressing, or gloved hand until an occlusive dressing can be applied.
  B. roller bandage.
  C. loose gauze dressing, or gloved hand until an occlusive dressing can be applied.
  D. piece of medical tape.

_____ **116.** If a patient's illness has existed over a long period of time or is recurring, it can be considered to be a/an _____ illness.
  A. acute
  B. chronic
  C. fatal
  D. generalized
  E. complaint

_____ **117.** Which of the following conditions can result in a behavioral emergency?
  A. Hypoxia
  B. Very low blood pressure
  C. Head trauma
  D. Excessive heat or cold
  E. All of the above.

_____ **118.** The **major** difference between heat exhaustion and heatstroke is:
  A. muscle cramping.
  B. the cessation of perspiration.
  C. shallow breathing.
  D. weakness.
  E. rapid pulse.

_____ **119.** Which of the following **is not** a potential cause of seizures?
  A. Chest pain
  B. Alcohol
  C. Fevers
  D. Brain tumors

_____ **120.** An infant's average pulse rate and respiratory rate is _____ when compared with pulse and respiratory rates in an adult.
  A. faster
  B. slower
  C. the same
  D. much slower

_____ **121.** Any situations that put you, patients, and bystanders in danger are called:
  A. emergencies.
  B. wreckage.
  C. hazards.
  D. alarms.

_____**122.** A first responder will be granted protection from civil liability if, while acting in good faith, providing care to the level of training to the **best** of their ability under the:
   A. Good Samaritan Law.
   B. Davis Act.
   C. Hold No Harm Statute.
   D. Myers Act.

_____**123.** Which of the following **is** **not** a way to combat stress?
   A. Eating a healthy diet
   B. Regular exercise
   C. Isolation
   D. Elimination or limitation of alcohol consumption
   E. Meditation

_____**124.** Which of the following is a warning sign of stress?
   A. Isolation
   B. Loss of appetite
   C. Problems sleeping
   D. Anxiety
   E. All of the above.

_____**125.** The five stages of the grieving process are denial, _____, bargaining, depression, and acceptance.
   A. solitude
   B. anxiety
   C. anger
   D. isolation
   E. annoyance

_____**126.** In the _____ phase of the grieving process, a person may refuse to accept the death or dying process.
   A. anger
   B. denial
   C. depression
   D. solitude
   E. acceptance

_____**127.** A special kind of stress encountered by emergency responders that results from their exposure to incidents of a critical nature is:
   A. pre-incident stress.
   B. personal stress.
   C. workplace stress.
   D. critical incident stress.

_____**128.** Critical incident stress debriefing (CISD) usually begins with a _____ that occurs a few hours after the critical incident and is short and informal.
   A. counseling session
   B. debriefing
   C. critique
   D. defusing
   E. team meeting

_____**129.** Which of the following **is not** an element of the Critical Incident Stress Management system?
   A. Leadership coaching
   B. Disaster support services
   C. On-scene support
   D. Community outreach programs
   E. Support for spouses and families

_____**130.** In the CISD process, a structured meeting called a _____ usually occurs within 24 to 72 hours after a critical incident.
   A. counseling session
   B. debriefing
   C. critique
   D. defusing
   E. team meeting

_____**131.** A type of incident that may cause a first responder to experience critical incident stress is one that involves:
   A. a multiple casualty incident or disaster.
   B. children.
   C. death or injury of a co-worker.
   D. All of the above.

_____**132.** All of the following are means of safeguarding your physical and emotional well-being **except**:
   A. ensuring scene safety.
   B. an annual psychological review.
   C. using universal precautions/including PPE.
   D. learning about stressors.

_____**133.** More healthcare workers die each year from _____ or its complications than from any other infectious disease.
   A. Human Immunodeficiency Virus (HIV)
   B. hepatitis B (HBV)
   C. Acquired Immune Deficiency Syndrome (AIDS)
   D. hepatitis C (HCV)

_____**134.** Trying to understand the feelings of the patient or family member is an example of:
   A. empathy.
   B. apathy.
   C. sympathy.
   D. tolerance.

_____**135.** _____ is/are a form of infection control based on the presumption that all body fluids are infectious.
A. Body substance isolation
B. Disease protocols
C. Universal protocols
D. Impermeable barriers

_____**136.** Difficulty sleeping, loss of appetite, and inability to concentrate are all warning signs of:
A. type A personality.
B. job burn-out.
C. diabetes.
D. stress.

_____**137.** All of the following are examples of infection control barriers **except**:
A. pocket face mask with one way valve.
B. eye shields.
C. nonrebreathing mask.
D. latex or vinyl gloves.

_____**138.** _____ are agents produced by the body to combat specific microorganisms.
A. Pathogens
B. Innoculations
C. Carriers
D. Antibodies

_____**139.** Needles used for intravenous access or injections **must** be disposed of in a:
A. regular waste container or trash receptacle.
B. biohazardous bag (red bag).
C. dumpster.
D. sharps container (hard plastic container).

_____**140.** What type of disease transmission is caused by touching a substance that contains an infectious agent?
A. Direct contact
B. Airborne transmission
C. Carrier-based
D. Vector-borne transmission

_____ **141.** A/An _____ is a special type of mask that filters out the smallest microorganisms in the air, including tuberculosis (TB).
A. pathogen
B. A44/BSI
C. N95/high efficiency particulate air (HEPA)
D. innoculation

_____**142.** The term for a person who has disease microorganisms in the body but <u>may</u> <u>not</u> have any symptoms of the disease is:
  A. transmitter.
  B. vector.
  C. carrier.
  D. pathogen.
  E. virulence.

_____**143.** After removing gloves and disposing of them properly, first responders should immediately:
  A. wash their hands.
  B. clean their equipment.
  C. find a new pair of gloves.
  D. wash their clothing.

_____**144.** A first responder <u>must</u> don a new pair of gloves:
  A. every shift.
  B. for each hour on duty.
  C. every week.
  D. for each patient contact.
  E. for every pediatric patient.

_____**145.** The <u>most</u> <u>effective</u> means of reducing risk of transmission of a disease is:
  A. cleaning with bleach.
  B. limiting patient contact.
  C. hand washing.
  D. making patients wear masks.

_____**146.** Which of the following is a potentially infectious body fluid?
  A. Blood
  B. Cerebrospinal fluid
  C. Vaginal discharge
  D. Semen
  E. All of the above.

_____**147.** _____ transmission occurs through direct or indirect contact with aerosolized particles suspended in air.
  A. Contact
  B. Airborne
  C. Vehicle
  D. Vector-borne
  E. Carrier-based

_____**148.** When washing the hands, after soap is applied, first responders must lather and scrub hands vigorously for at least _____ seconds.
  A. 30
  B. 45
  C. 5
  D. 60
  E. 15

_____**149.** What kind of disease transmission has occurred when a person receives disease from an insect bite?
  A. Contact transmission
  B. Airborne transmission
  C. Carrier-based transmission
  D. Vector-borne transmission

_____**150.** Appropriate body substances isolation (BSI) precautions should be taken for:
  A. every patient.
  B. patients with hepatitis B.
  C. adult patients.
  D. patients who are bleeding.
  E. patients who are coughing.

Did you score higher than 80 percent on Examination I-3? Circle Yes or No in ink.

Feedback Step

Now, what do we do with your "yes" and "no" answers given throughout the SAEP process? First, return to any response that has "no" circled. Go back to the highlighted answers for those examination items missed. Read and study the paragraph preceding the location of the answer as well as the paragraph following the paragraph where the answer is located. This will expand your knowledge base for the missed question, put it in a broader perspective, and improve associative learning. Remember, you are trying to develop mastery of the required knowledge. Scoring 80 percent on an examination is good, but it is not mastery performance. To be at the top of your group, you must score much higher than 80 percent on your training, promotion, or certification examination.

Carefully review the Summary of Key Rules for Taking an Examination and Summary of Helpful Hints on the next two pages. Do this review now and at least two additional times prior to taking your next examination.

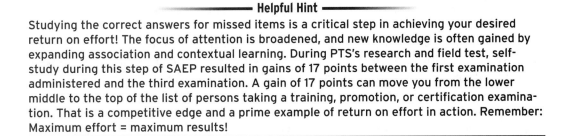

Helpful Hint

Studying the correct answers for missed items is a critical step in achieving your desired return on effort! The focus of attention is broadened, and new knowledge is often gained by expanding association and contextual learning. During PTS's research and field test, self-study during this step of SAEP resulted in gains of 17 points between the first examination administered and the third examination. A gain of 17 points can move you from the lower middle to the top of the list of persons taking a training, promotion, or certification examination. That is a competitive edge and a prime example of return on effort in action. Remember: Maximum effort = maximum results!

Summary of Key Rules for Taking an Examination

Rule 1—Examination preparation is not easy. Preparation is 95% perspiration and 5% inspiration.

Rule 2—Follow the steps very carefully. Do not try to reinvent or shortcut the system. It really works just as it was designed to!

Rule 3—Mark with an "X" any examination items for which you guessed the answer. For maximum return on effort, you should also research any answer that you guessed even if you guessed correctly. Find the correct answer, highlight it, and then read the entire paragraph that contains the answer. Be honest and mark all questions on which you guessed. Some examinations have a correction for guessing built into the scoring process. The correction for guessing can reduce your final examination score. If you are guessing, you are not mastering the material.

Rule 4—Read questions twice if you have any misunderstanding, especially if the question contains complex directions or activities.

Rule 5—If you want someone to perform effectively and efficiently on the job, the training and testing program must be aligned to achieve this result.

Rule 6—When preparing examination items for job-specific requirements, the writer must be a subject matter expert with current experience at the level that the technical information is applied.

Rule 7—Good luck = good preparation.

Summary of Helpful Hints

<u>Helpful Hint</u>—Most of the time your first impression is the best. More than 41% of changed answers during PTS's SAEP field test were changed from a right answer to a wrong answer. Another 33% were changed from a wrong answer to another wrong answer. Only 26% of answers were changed from wrong to right. In fact three participants did not make a perfect score of 100% because they changed one right answer to a wrong one! Think twice before you change your answer. The odds are not in your favor.

<u>Helpful Hint</u>—Researching correct answers is one of the most important activities in SAEP. Locate the correct answer for all missed examination items. Highlight the correct answer. Then read the entire paragraph containing the answer. This will put the answer in context for you and provide important learning by association.

<u>Helpful Hint</u>—Proceed through all missed examination items using the same technique. Reading the entire paragraph improves retention of the information and helps you develop an association with the material and learn the correct answers. This step may sound simple. A major finding during the development and field testing of SAEP was that you learn from your mistakes.

<u>Helpful Hint</u>—Follow each step carefully to realize the best return on effort. Would you consider investing your money in a venture without some chance of earning a return on that investment? Examination preparation is no different. You are investing time and expecting a significant return for that time. If, indeed, time is money, then you are investing money and are due a return on that investment. Doing things right and doing the right things in examination preparation will ensure the maximum return on effort.

<u>Helpful Hint</u>—Try to determine why you selected the wrong answer. Usually something influenced your selection. Focus on the difference between your wrong answer and the correct answer. Carefully read and study the entire paragraph containing the correct answer. Highlight the answer.

<u>Helpful Hint</u>—Studying the correct answers for missed items is a critical step in achieving your desired return on effort! The focus of attention is broadened, and new knowledge is often gained by expanding association and contextual learning. During PTS's research and field test, self-study during this step of SAEP resulted in gains of 17 points between the first examination administered and the third examination. A gain of 17 points can move you from the lower middle to the top of the list of persons taking a training, promotion, or certification examination. That is a competitive edge and a prime example of return on effort in action. Remember: Maximum effort = maximum results!

PHASE II

How Examination Developers Think–Getting Inside Their Heads

Now that you've finished the examination practice, this phase will assist you in understanding and applying examination-taking skills. Developing your knowledge of how examination professionals think and prepare examinations is not cheating. Most serious examination takers have spent many hours reviewing various examinations to gain an insight into the technology used to develop them. It is a demanding technology when used properly. You probably already know this if you have prepared examination items and administered them in your fire department.

Phase II will not cover all the ways and means of examination-item writing. Examination-item writers use far too many techniques to cover adequately in this book. Instead, the focus here is on key techniques that will help you achieve a better score on your examination.

How are examination items derived?

Professional examination-item writers use three basic techniques to derive examination items from text or technical reference materials: verbatim, deduction, and inference.

The most common technique is to take examination items verbatim from materials in the reference list. This technique doesn't work well for mastering information, however. The verbatim form of testing encourages rote learning—that is, simply memorizing the material. The results of this type of learning are not long-lasting, nor are they appropriate for learning and retaining the critical knowledge that you must have for on-the-job performance. Consequently, SAEP doesn't create the majority of examination questions covering the National Standard Curriculum using the verbatim technique.

Professional examination-item writers tend to use verbatim testing at the very basic level of job classifications. A first responder, for instance, is expected to learn many basic facts. At this level, verbatim examination items can be justified.

In the higher ranks of Emergency Medical Services other methods are more beneficial and productive for mastering higher cognitive knowledge and skills. At the higher cognitive levels of an occupation, such as EMS supervisor, examination development will therefore rely on other means. The most important technique at the higher cognitive levels is using deduction as the basis for examination items. This technique requires logic and analytical skills and often requires the examination taker to read materials several times to answer the examination item. It is not, then, a matter of simply repeating the information that results in a verbatim answer.

At the first responder level, most activities are carefully supervised by a more experienced technician or company officer. At this level, the responder is expected to closely follow commands and is encouraged not to use deductive reasoning that can lead to "freelance" responder tactics. As one progresses to a higher level job and gains experience, deductive reasoning and inferences skills are developed and applied. Most of these skills are related to personal safety and the safety of those on the scene. Most size-up and strategies are developed and passed from the officers on the scene to the first responders.

━━━━━━━━━━━━ **Rule 5** ━━━━━━━━━━━━

If you want someone to perform effectively and efficiently on the job, the training and testing program must be aligned to achieve this result.

Rule #5 is paramount for first responders. Effective and efficient first responders are able to receive incident commands, follow instructions, and perform their tasks as safely and as rapidly as they can. There are limited opportunities for first responders to do much else, because they serve as the first line of action at the emergency scene.

Consider the following example of deductive reasoning: an incident call is received from the telecommunicator stating that an infant has a high temperature and is convulsing. Just this amount of information should cause the first responder to immediately plan the response, conduct size-up activities, and review infant care procedures en route. Some of these deductive responses will have you focus on the infant's age, past medical history, location, access, and many other possible factors. If you have an EMT or Paramedic background, a list of several items could be deduced that would expedite an efficient and effective response to the incident.

You can probably think of many first responder tasks and circumstances that rely on deductive reasoning. The more experience you gain on the emergency scene as a medical first responder, the more often you will be called upon to practice deductive reasoning and inference from emergency data, and the more efficient and effective you will become, whether the situation involves clearing an airway or attending to the emergency needs of an infant.

Legendary football coach Vince Lombardi was once asked about the precision performance of his offensive and defensive teams. It was suggested that Lombardi must spend a lot of time on the practice field to achieve those results. Lombardi responded, "Practice doesn't make perfect; only perfect practice makes perfect." This is exactly what is required to be an outstanding examination taker. Most people don't perfectly practice examination-taking skills.

A third technique used by professional examination-item writers is to rely on inference or implied answers to develop examination items. Inference requires contrasting, comparing, analyzing, evaluating, and other high-level cognitive skills. Tables, charts, graphs, and other instruments for presenting data provide excellent means for deriving inference-based examination items. Implied answers are based on logic. They rely on your ability to use logical processes or series of facts to arrive at a plausible answer.

For example, recent data gathered by the NFPA stated that heart attacks remain the leading cause of death for fire service personnel. Other NFPA-supplied data indicated that strains and sprains are the leading cause of injuries on the job. Several inferences can be made from these relatively simple statements. A safety officer can infer the results of the NFPA study to his or her own personnel and use the information as a trigger for checking on personnel, conducting surveys, reviewing accident records, and comparing the study results with actual experience. Is that particular EMS Division doing better or worse in terms of these important health issues? Are the first responders getting the right exercise? Are they diligent in keeping the vehicles, facilities, and emergency scene free from the activities that may lead to strains and sprains? The basic inference here is that any particular organization may be similar or different in some ways from the generalized data.

Sometimes it may be difficult to find an answer to an examination item because it is measuring your ability to make deductions and draw inferences from the technical materials.

How are examination items written and validated?

Once the pertinent information is identified and the technique for writing an examination item selected, the professional examination-item writer will prepare a draft. The draft examination item is then referenced to specific technical information, such as a textbook, manufacturer's manual, or other related technical information. If the information is derived from a job-based requirement, then it should also be validated by job incumbents (i.e., those who are actually performing in the occupation at the specific level of the required knowledge).

━━━━━━━━ **Rule 6** ━━━━━━━━

When preparing examination items for job-specific requirements, the writer must be a subject matter expert with current experience at the level where the technical information is applied.

Rule #6 ensures that the examination item has a basic level of job content validity. The final level of job content validity is determined by using committees or surveys of job incumbents who certify the information to be current and required on the job. The information must be in a category of "need to know" or "must know" to be considered job relevant. The technical information must be accurate. Because subject matter experts do need basic training in examination-item writing, it is recommended that a professional in examination technology be part of the review process so that basic rules and guidelines of the industry are followed.

Finally, the examination items must be field tested. Once this testing is complete, statistical and analytical tools are available to help revise and improve the examination items. These techniques and tools go well beyond the scope of this *Exam Prep* book. Professionals are available to conduct these data analyses, and their services should be used.

Good Practices in Examination-Item and Examination Development

The most reliable examinations are objective. That is, each question has only one answer that is accepted by members of the occupation. This objective quality permits fair and equitable examinations. The most popular types of objective examination items are multiple choice, true/false, matching, and completion (fill in the blanks).

Valid and reliable job-relevant examinations for the Emergency Medical Service industry must satisfy 10 rules:

1. They do not contain trick questions.
2. They are short and easy to read, using language and terms appropriate to the target examination population.
3. They are supported with technical references, validation information, and data on their difficulty, discrimination, and other item analysis statistics.
4. They are formatted to meet recognized testing standards and examples.
5. They focus on the "need to know" and "must know" aspects of the job.
6. They are fair and objective.
7. They are not based on obscure and trivial knowledge and skills.
8. They can be easily defended in terms of job-content requirements.
9. They meet national and other professional job qualification standards.
10. They demonstrate their usefulness as part of a comprehensive testing program, including written, oral, and performance examination items.

The primary challenges of job-relevant examinations relate to their currency and validity. Careful recording of data, technical reference sources, and the examination writer's qualifications are important. Examinations that affect someone's ability to be promoted, certified, or licensed, as well as to complete training that leads to a job, have exacting requirements both in published documents and in the laws of the land.

Three Common Myths of Examination Construction

1. **Myth:** If in doubt about the answer for a multiple-choice examination item, select the longest answer.

   Reality: Professional examination-item writers use short answers as correct ones at an equal or higher percentage than longer answers. Remember, there are usually choices A–D. That leaves three other possibilities for the correct answer other than the longest one. Statistically speaking, the longest answer is less likely to be correct.

2. **Myth:** If in doubt about the answer for a multiple-choice examination item, select "C".

   Reality: Computer technology and examination-item banking permit multiple versions of examinations to be developed simultaneously. This is typically achieved by moving the correct answer to different locations (for example, version 1 will have the correct answer in the "C" position, version 2 will have it in the "D" position, and so forth).

3. **Myth:** Watch for errors in singular examination-item stems with plural choices in the A–D answers, or vice versa.

   Reality: Most computer-based programs have spelling and grammar checking utilities. If this mistake occurs, an editing error is the probable cause and usually has nothing to do with detecting the right answer.

Some Things That Work

1. Two to three days before your examination, review the examination items you missed in SAEP. Read those highlighted answers and the entire paragraph one more time.
2. During the examination, carefully read each examination item twice. Once you have selected your answer, read the examination item and answer together. This technique can prompt you to recall information that you studied during your examination preparation activities.
3. Apply what you learned in SAEP. Eliminate as many distracters as possible to improve your chance of answering the question correctly.
4. Pace yourself. Know how much time you have to take the examination. If an examination item is requiring too much time, write its number down and continue with the next examination item. Often, a later examination item will trigger your memory and make the earlier examination item seem easier to answer. (For a time pacing strategy, see the Examination Pacing Table at the end of Phase III.)
5. Don't panic if you don't know some examination items. Leave them to answer later. The most important thing is to finish the examination, because there may be several examination items at the end of the examination that you do know.
6. As time runs out for taking the examination, do not panic. Concentrate on answering those difficult examination items that you skipped.
7. Double-check your answer sheets to make sure you have not accidentally left an answer blank.

8. Once you complete the examination, return to the difficult examination items. Often, while taking an examination, other examination items will cause you to remember or associate those answers with the difficult examination-item answers. The longer the examination, the more likely you will be to gather the information needed to answer more difficult examination items.

There are many other helpful hints that can be used to improve your examination-taking skills. If you want to research the materials on how to take examinations and raise your final score, visit your local library, a bookstore, or the Web for additional resources. The main reason we developed SAEP is to provide practice and help you develop examination-taking skills that you can use throughout your life.

PHASE III

The Basics of Mental and Physical Preparation

Mental Preparation—I Can Get My Head Ready!

The two most common mental blocks to examination taking are examination anxiety and fear of failure. In the Fire and Emergency Medical Service, these feelings can create significant performance barriers. Overcoming severe conditions may require some professional psychological assistance, which is beyond the scope of this *Exam Prep* book.

The root cause of examination anxiety and fear of failure is often lack of self-confidence. SAEP was designed to help improve your self-confidence by providing evidence of your mastery of the material on the examination. Look at your scores as you progress through Phase I. Review your Personal Progress Plotter; it will help you gain confidence in your knowledge of the first responder curriculum. Look at your Personal Progress Plotter the day before your scheduled examination and experience renewed confidence.

Let's examine the meaning of anxiety. Knowing what it is will help you deal with it at examination time. According to *Webster's Dictionary,* anxiety is "uneasiness and distress about future uncertainties." Many of us have real anxiety about taking examinations, and it is a natural response for some, often prefaced by questions like these: Am I ready for this? Do I have a good idea of what will be on the examination? Will I make the lowest score? Will John Doe score higher than me?

These questions and concerns are normal. Remember that hundreds of people have gone through SAEP and achieved an average gain of 17 points in their scores. The preparation process will help you maintain your self-confidence. Once again, review the evidence in your Personal Progress Plotter to see what you have accomplished.

Fear, according to *Webster's Dictionary,* is "alarm and agitation caused by the expectation or realization of danger." It is a normal reaction to examinations. To deal with it, first analyze the degree of fear you may be experiencing several days before the examination date. Then focus on the positive experiences you had as you finished SAEP. Putting your fear in perspective by using positives to eliminate or minimize it is a very important examination-taking skill. The more you focus on your positive accomplishments in mastering the materials, the less fear you will experience.

If your fear and anxiety persist even after you take steps to build your confidence, you may want to get some professional assistance. Do it now! Don't wait until the week before the examination. There may be real issues that a professional can help you deal with to overcome these feelings. Hypnosis and other forms of treatment have been found to be very helpful. Consult with an expert in this area.

Physical Preparation—Am I Really Ready?

Physical preparation is the element that is probably most ignored in examination preparation. In the Emergency Medical Service, examinations are often given at locations away from home. If this is the case, you need to be especially careful of key physical concerns. More will be said about that later.

In general, following these helpful hints will help you concentrate, enhance your examination performance, and add points to your score.

1. Do not "cram" for the examination. This factor was found to be first in importance during PTS's field test of SAEP. Cramming results in examination anxiety, adds to confusion, and tends to lessen the effectiveness of the examination-taking skills you already possess. Avoid cramming!

2. Get a normal night's rest. It may even be wise to take a day off before the examination to rest. Do not schedule an all-night shift right before your examination.

3. Avoid taking excessive stimulants or medications that inhibit your thinking processes. Eat at least three well-balanced meals before the day of the examination. It is a good practice to carry a balanced energy bar (not candy) and a bottle of water into the examination area. Examination anxiety and fear can cause a dry mouth, which can lead to further aggravation. Nibbling on the energy bar also has a settling effect and supplies some "brain food."

4. If the examination is taking place at an out-of-town location, do the following:
   - Avoid a "night out with friends." Lack of rest, partying, and fatigue are major examination performance killers.
   - Check your room carefully. Eliminate things that may aggravate you, interfere with your rest, or cause any discomfort. If the mattress isn't good, the pillows are horrible, or the room has an unpleasant odor, change rooms or even hotels.
   - Wake up in plenty of time to take a relaxing shower or soaking bath. Don't put yourself in a "rush" mode. Things should be carefully planned so that you arrive at the examination site ahead of time, calm, and collected.

5. Listen to the examination proctor. The proctor usually has rules that you must follow. Important instructions and directions are usually given. Ask clarifying questions immediately and listen to the responses to questions raised by the other examination takers. Most examination environments are carefully controlled and may not permit questions you raise that are covered in the proctor's comments or deal with the technical content in the examination itself. Be attentive, focus, and succeed.

6. Remain calm and breathe. Pace yourself. Apply your examination-taking skills learned during SAEP.

7. Remember the analogy of an examination as a competitive event. If you want to gain a competitive edge, carefully follow all phases of SAEP. This process has yielded outstanding results in the past and will do so for you.

Time Management During Examinations

The following table will help you pace yourself during an examination. You should become familiar with the table and be able to construct your own when you are in the examination room and getting ready to start the examination process. This effort will take a few minutes, but it will make a tremendous contribution to your time management during the examination.

Here is how the table works. First you divide the examination time into 6 equal parts. If you have 3.5 hours (210 minutes) for the examination, then each of the six time parts contains 35 minutes (210 ÷ 6 = 35 minutes). Now divide the number of examination items by 5. For example, if the examination has 150 examination items, 150 ÷ 5 = 30. Now, with the math done, we can set up a table that tells you approximately how many examination items you should answer in 35 minutes (the equal time divisions). You should be on or near examination item 30 at the end of the first 35 minutes and so forth. Notice that we divided the number of examination items by 5 and the time available by 6. The extra time block of 35 minutes is used to double-check your answer sheet, focus on difficult questions, and calm your nerves. This technique will work wonders for your stress level, and yes, it will improve your examination score.

Examination Pacing Table

Time for Examination	Minutes for 6 Equal Time Parts	Number of Examination Items	Examination Items per Time Part	Time for Examination Review
210 minutes (3.5 hours)	35 minutes	150	30 (number of examination items to be answered)	35 minutes (chilling and double-checking examination)
150 minutes (2.5 hours)	25 minutes	100	20 (number of examination items to be answered)	25 minutes (chilling and double-checking examination)

The Examination Pacing Table can be altered by adjusting the time and examination item variables, as either may change in the real examination environment. For instance, if the time changes, adjust the amount of time available to answer the examination items in each of the five time blocks. If the examination item numbers increase or decrease, adjust the number of examination items to be answered in the time blocks.

Take some precautions when using this time management strategy:

1. Do not panic if you run a few minutes behind in each time block. This time management strategy should not stress you while you are using it. Most people tend to pick up their pace as they move into the examination.
2. During the examination, carefully mark or note examination items that you need to return to during your review time block. This will help you expedite your examination completion check.
3. Do not be afraid to ask for more time to complete your examination. In most cases, the time limit is flexible or should be.
4. Double-check your answer sheet to make sure that you didn't leave blank responses and that you didn't double-mark answers. Double-markings are most often counted as wrong answers. Make sure that any erasures are made cleanly. Caution: When you change your answer, make sure that you really want to do so. The odds are not in your favor unless something on the examination really influenced the change.

APPENDIX A

Examination I-1 Answer Key

Directions

Follow these steps carefully for completing the feedback part of SAEP:

1. After calculating your score, look up the answers for the examination items you missed as well as those on which you guessed, even if you guessed correctly. If you are guessing, it means the answer is not perfectly clear. In this process, we are committed to making you as knowledgeable as possible.

2. Enter the number of missed and guessed examination items in the blanks on your Personal Progress Plotter.

3. Highlight the answer in the reference materials. Read the paragraph preceding and the paragraph following the one in which the correct answer is located. Enter the paragraph number and page number next to the guessed or missed examination item on your examination. Count any part of a paragraph at the beginning of the page as one paragraph until you reach the paragraph containing your highlighted answer. This step will help you locate and review your missed and guessed examination items later in the process. It is essential to learning the material in context and by association. These learning techniques (context/association) are the very backbone of the SAEP approach.

4. Once you have completed the feedback part, you may proceed to the next examination.

1. Reference: NFPA 1001, 4.3
   Brady, *First Responder*, 7th Edition, 1st Printing, page 507.
   Answer: D

2. Reference: NFPA 1001, 4.3
   Brady, *First Responder*, 7th Edition, 1st Printing, pages 505 and 507.
   Delmar, *First Responder Handbook*, Fire Service Edition, page 333.
   Mosby, *Emergency First Responder, Making the Difference*, 1st Edition, page 348.
   Jones and Bartlett, AAOS, *First Responder, Your First Response in Emergency Care*, 3rd Edition, page 390.
   Answer: C

3. Reference: NFPA 1001, 4.3
   Brady, *First Responder*, 7th Edition, 1st Printing, page 514.
   Answer: B

4. Reference: NFPA 1001, 4.3
   Brady, *First Responder*, 7th Edition, 1st Printing, page 515.
   Answer: D

5. Reference: NFPA 1001, 4.3

Brady, *First Responder*, 7th Edition, 1st Printing, page 550.

Delmar, *First Responder Handbook*, Fire Service Edition, pages 272 and 276.

Mosby, *Emergency First Responder, Making the Difference*, 1st Edition, page 347.

Jones and Bartlett, AAOS, *First Responder, Your First Response in Emergency Care*, 3rd Edition, page 394.

Answer: A

6. Reference: NFPA 1001, 4.3

Brady, *First Responder*, 7th Edition, 1st Printing, pages 98 and 99.

Delmar, *First Responder Handbook*, Fire Service Edition, pages 125–127.

Mosby, *Emergency First Responder, Making the Difference*, 1st Edition, pages 106 and 107.

Jones and Bartlett, AAOS, *First Responder, Your First Response in Emergency Care*, 3rd Edition, pages 103 and 104.

Answer: A

7. Reference: NFPA 1001, 4.3

Brady, *First Responder*, 7th Edition, 1st Printing, pages 98 and 99.

Delmar, *First Responder Handbook*, Fire Service Edition, page 125.

Mosby, *Emergency First Responder, Making the Difference*, 1st Edition, page 106.

Jones and Bartlett, AAOS, *First Responder, Your First Response in Emergency Care*, 3rd Edition, page 104.

Answer: C

8. Reference: NFPA 1001, 4.3

Brady, *First Responder*, 7th Edition, 1st Printing, page 100.

Delmar, *First Responder Handbook*, Fire Service Edition, page 127.

Mosby, *Emergency First Responder, Making the Difference,* 1st Edition, pages 61–63 and 106.

Jones and Bartlett, AAOS, *First Responder, Your First Response in Emergency Care*, 3rd Edition, page 104.

Answer: D

9. Reference: NFPA 1001, 4.3

Brady, *First Responder*, 7th Edition, 1st Printing, pages 102 and 111.

Delmar, *First Responder Handbook*, Fire Service Edition, pages 131–132.

Mosby, *Emergency First Responder, Making the Difference*, 1st Edition, page 109.

Jones and Bartlett, AAOS, *First Responder, Your First Response in Emergency Care*, 3rd Edition, page 107.

Answer: B

10. Reference: NFPA 1001, 4.3

Brady, *First Responder*, 7th Edition, 1st Printing, page 121.

Delmar, *First Responder Handbook*, Fire Service Edition, page 138.

Mosby, *Emergency First Responder, Making the Difference*, 1st Edition, page 109.

Jones and Bartlett, AAOS, *First Responder, Your First Response in Emergency Care*, 3rd Edition, page 109.

Answer: C

11. Reference: NFPA 1001, 4.3

Brady, *First Responder*, 7th Edition, 1st Printing, pages 548 and 558.

Delmar, *First Responder Handbook*, Fire Service Edition, pages 140–141.

Mosby, *Emergency First Responder, Making the Difference*, 1st Edition, pages 116 and 127.

Jones and Bartlett, AAOS, *First Responder, Your First Response in Emergency Care*, 3rd Edition, pages 117 and 443.

Answer: E

12. Reference: NFPA 1001, 4.3

Brady, *First Responder*, 7th Edition, 1st Printing, pages 548 and 558.

Delmar, *First Responder Handbook*, Fire Service Edition, page 141.

Mosby, *Emergency First Responder, Making the Difference*, 1st Edition, page 128.

Jones and Bartlett, AAOS, *First Responder, Your First Response in Emergency Care*, 3rd Edition, page 446.

Answer: A

13. Reference: NFPA 1001, 4.3

Brady, *First Responder*, 7th Edition, 1st Printing, page 128.

Delmar, *First Responder Handbook*, Fire Service Edition, page 146.

Mosby, *Emergency First Responder, Making the Difference*, 1st Edition, page 111.

Jones and Bartlett, AAOS, *First Responder, Your First Response in Emergency Care*, 3rd Edition, page 112.

Answer: C

14. Reference: NFPA 1001, 4.3

Brady, *First Responder*, 7th Edition, 1st Printing, page 554.

Delmar, *First Responder Handbook*, Fire Service Edition, page 150.

Mosby, *Emergency First Responder, Making the Difference*, 1st Edition, pages 126 and 132.

Jones and Bartlett, AAOS, *First Responder, Your First Response in Emergency Care*, 3rd Edition, page 442.

Answer: D

15. Reference: NFPA 1001, 4.3

Brady, *First Responder*, 7th Edition, 1st Printing, pages 442 and 554.

Delmar, *First Responder Handbook*, Fire Service Edition, page 150.

Mosby, *Emergency First Responder, Making the Difference*, 1st Edition, page 126.

Jones and Bartlett, AAOS, *First Responder, Your First Response in Emergency Care*, 3rd Edition, page 442.

Answer: C

16. Reference: NFPA 1001, 4.3

Brady, *First Responder*, 7th Edition, 1st Printing, page 285.

Delmar, *First Responder Handbook*, Fire Service Edition, pages 186–188.

Mosby, *Emergency First Responder, Making the Difference*, 1st Edition, page 64.

Jones and Bartlett, AAOS, *First Responder, Your First Response in Emergency Care*, 3rd Edition, page 55.

Answer: C

17. Reference: NFPA 1001, 4.3
Brady, *First Responder*, 7th Edition, 1st Printing, page 285.
Delmar, *First Responder Handbook*, Fire Service Edition, page 195.
Jones and Bartlett, AAOS, *First Responder, Your First Response in Emergency Care*, 3rd Edition, page 259.
Answer: A

18. Reference: NFPA 1001, 4.3
Brady, *First Responder*, 7th Edition, 1st Printing, page 289.
Delmar, *First Responder Handbook*, Fire Service Edition, page 167.
Mosby, *Emergency First Responder, Making the Difference*, 1st Edition, pages 240, 241, and 243.
Jones and Bartlett, AAOS, *First Responder, Your First Response in Emergency Care*, 3rd Edition, page 264.
Answer: C

19. Reference: NFPA 1001, 4.3
Brady, *First Responder*, 7th Edition, 1st Printing, page 292.
Mosby, *Emergency First Responder, Making the Difference*, 1st Edition, page 241.
Answer: B

20. Reference: NFPA 1001, 4.3
Brady, *First Responder*, 7th Edition, 1st Printing, page 293.
Delmar, *First Responder Handbook*, Fire Service Edition, page 238.
Mosby, *Emergency First Responder, Making the Difference*, 1st Edition, pages 241 and 242.
Jones and Bartlett, AAOS, *First Responder, Your First Response in Emergency Care*, 3rd Edition, page 265.
Answer: C

21. Reference: NFPA 1001, 4.3
Brady, *First Responder*, 7th Edition, 1st Printing, pages 289–297.
Delmar, *First Responder Handbook*, Fire Service Edition, pages 237–238.
Mosby, *Emergency First Responder, Making the Difference*, 1st Edition, pages 240–241.
Jones and Bartlett, AAOS, *First Responder, Your First Response in Emergency Care*, 3rd Edition, pages 265 and 269.
Answer: A

22. Reference: NFPA 1001, 4.3
Brady, *First Responder*, 7th Edition, 1st Printing, page 302.
Mosby, *Emergency First Responder, Making the Difference*, 1st Edition, page 141.
Jones and Bartlett, AAOS, *First Responder, Your First Response in Emergency Care*, 3rd Edition, page 275.
Answer: D

23. Reference: NFPA 1001, 4.3
Brady, *First Responder*, 7th Edition, 1st Printing, page 316.
Mosby, *Emergency First Responder, Making the Difference*, 1st Edition, pages 247 and 248.
Jones and Bartlett, AAOS, *First Responder, Your First Response in Emergency Care*, 3rd Edition, page 267.
Answer: C

24. Reference: NFPA 1001, 4.3

Brady, *First Responder*, 7th Edition, 1st Printing, page 422.

Delmar, *First Responder Handbook*, Fire Service Edition, pages 309 and 311.

Mosby, *Emergency First Responder, Making the Difference*, 1st Edition, page 294.

Jones and Bartlett, AAOS, *First Responder, Your First Response in Emergency Care*, 3rd Edition, page 330.

Answer: D

25. Reference: NFPA 1001, 4.3

Brady, *First Responder*, 7th Edition, 1st Printing, page 422.

Mosby, *Emergency First Responder, Making the Difference*, 1st Edition, page 294.

Answer: C

26. Reference: NFPA 1001, 4.3

Brady, *First Responder*, 7th Edition, 1st Printing, page 424.

Jones and Bartlett, AAOS, *First Responder, Your First Response in Emergency Care*, 3rd Edition, page 333.

Answer: B

27. Reference: NFPA 1001, 4.3

Brady, *First Responder*, 7th Edition, 1st Printing, page 424.

Mosby, *Emergency First Responder, Making the Difference*, 1st Edition, page 295.

Jones and Bartlett, AAOS, *First Responder, Your First Response in Emergency Care*, 3rd Edition, page 333.

Answer: C

28. Reference: NFPA 1001, 4.3

Brady, *First Responder*, 7th Edition, 1st Printing, pages 425–428.

Mosby, *Emergency First Responder, Making the Difference*, 1st Edition, page 299.

Answer: B

29. Reference: NFPA 1001, 4.3

Brady, *First Responder*, 7th Edition, 1st Printing, page 423.

Mosby, *Emergency First Responder, Making the Difference*, 1st Edition, page 301.

Jones and Bartlett, AAOS, *First Responder, Your First Response in Emergency Care*, 3rd Edition, page 341.

Answer: B

30. Reference: NFPA 1001, 4.3

Brady, *First Responder*, 7th Edition, 1st Printing, pages 104 and 194.

Delmar, *First Responder Handbook*, Fire Service Edition, page 143.

Mosby, *Emergency First Responder, Making the Difference*, 1st Edition, pages 147 and 185.

Jones and Bartlett, AAOS, *First Responder, Your First Response in Emergency Care*, 3rd Edition, page 183.

Answer: D

31. Reference: NFPA 1001, 4.3

Brady, *First Responder*, 7th Edition, 1st Printing, page 184.

Delmar, *First Responder Handbook*, Fire Service Edition, page 205.

Mosby, *Emergency First Responder, Making the Difference*, 1st Edition, pages 181, 183, and 204.

Jones and Bartlett, AAOS, *First Responder, Your First Response in Emergency Care*, 3rd Edition, page 447.

Answer: D

32. Reference: NFPA 1001, 4.3

Brady, *First Responder*, 7th Edition, 1st Printing, page 209.

Delmar, *First Responder Handbook*, Fire Service Edition, page 207.

Mosby, *Emergency First Responder, Making the Difference*, 1st Edition, page 197.

Jones and Bartlett, AAOS, *First Responder, Your First Response in Emergency Care*, 3rd Edition, page 447.

Answer: D

33. Reference: NFPA 1001, 4.3

Delmar, *First Responder Handbook*, Fire Service Edition, page 207.

Mosby, *Emergency First Responder, Making the Difference*, 1st Edition, page 199.

Jones and Bartlett, AAOS, *First Responder, Your First Response in Emergency Care*, 3rd Edition, page 447.

Answer: A

34. Reference: NFPA 1001, 4.3

Brady, *First Responder*, 7th Edition, 1st Printing, page 204.

Delmar, *First Responder Handbook*, Fire Service Edition, page 210.

Answer: C

35. Reference: NFPA 1001, 4.3

Brady, *First Responder*, 7th Edition, 1st Printing, pages 206–207.

Delmar, *First Responder Handbook*, Fire Service Edition, page 210.

Mosby, *Emergency First Responder, Making the Difference*, 1st Edition, page 182.

Jones and Bartlett, AAOS, *First Responder, Your First Response in Emergency Care*, 3rd Edition, page 446.

Answer: B

36. Reference: NFPA 1001, 4.3

Brady, *First Responder*, 7th Edition, 1st Printing, page 207.

Delmar, *First Responder Handbook*, Fire Service Edition, page 211.

Mosby, *Emergency First Responder, Making the Difference*, 1st Edition, pages 199 and 200.

Jones and Bartlett, AAOS, *First Responder, Your First Response in Emergency Care*, 3rd Edition, page 449.

Answer: A

37. Reference: NFPA 1001, 4.3

Brady, *First Responder*, 7th Edition, 1st Printing, page 206.

Delmar, *First Responder Handbook*, Fire Service Edition, page 212.

Mosby, *Emergency First Responder, Making the Difference*, 1st Edition, pages 199 and 200.

Jones and Bartlett, AAOS, *First Responder, Your First Response in Emergency Care*, 3rd Edition, page 448.

Answer: C

38. Reference: NFPA 1001, 4.3

Brady, *First Responder*, 7th Edition, 1st Printing, page 206.

Delmar, *First Responder Handbook*, Fire Service Edition, page 213.

Mosby, *Emergency First Responder, Making the Difference*, 1st Edition, page 198.

Answer: B

39. Reference: NFPA 1001, 4.3

Brady, *First Responder*, 7th Edition, 1st Printing, page 207.

Delmar, *First Responder Handbook*, Fire Service Edition, page 207.

Mosby, *Emergency First Responder, Making the Difference*, 1st Edition, page 198.

Jones and Bartlett, AAOS, *First Responder, Your First Response in Emergency Care*, 3rd Edition, page 449.

Answer: B

40. Reference: NFPA 1001, 4.3

Brady, *First Responder*, 7th Edition, 1st Printing, page 185.

Delmar, *First Responder Handbook*, Fire Service Edition, page 193.

Mosby, *Emergency First Responder, Making the Difference*, 1st Edition, page 180.

Jones and Bartlett, AAOS, *First Responder, Your First Response in Emergency Care*, 3rd Edition, page 176.

Answer: A

41. Reference: NFPA 1001, 4.3

Brady, *First Responder*, 7th Edition, 1st Printing, page 57.

Delmar, *First Responder Handbook*, Fire Service Edition, page 72.

Answer: A

42. Reference: NFPA 1001, 4.3

Brady, *First Responder*, 7th Edition, 1st Printing, page 55.

Delmar, *First Responder Handbook*, Fire Service Edition, page 72.

Mosby, *Emergency First Responder, Making the Difference*, 1st Edition, pages 58–59.

Jones and Bartlett, AAOS, *First Responder, Your First Response in Emergency Care*, 3rd Edition, page 51.

Answer: D

43. Reference: NFPA 1001, 4.3

Brady, *First Responder*, 7th Edition, 1st Printing, page 58.

Delmar, *First Responder Handbook*, Fire Service Edition, page 73.

Mosby, *Emergency First Responder, Making the Difference*, 1st Edition, page 69.

Jones and Bartlett, AAOS, *First Responder, Your First Response in Emergency Care*, 3rd Edition, page 56.

Answer: C

44. Reference: NFPA 1001, 4.3

Brady, *First Responder*, 7th Edition, 1st Printing, page 60.

Delmar, *First Responder Handbook*, Fire Service Edition, page 172.

Mosby, *Emergency First Responder, Making the Difference*, 1st Edition, pages 61 and 159.

Answer: C

45. Reference: NFPA 1001, 4.3

Brady, *First Responder*, 7th Edition, 1st Printing, page 62.

Delmar, *First Responder Handbook*, Fire Service Edition, page 76.

Mosby, *Emergency First Responder, Making the Difference*, 1st Edition, page 69.

Jones and Bartlett, AAOS, *First Responder, Your First Response in Emergency Care*, 3rd Edition, page 59.

Answer: C

46. Reference: NFPA 1001, 4.3

Brady, *First Responder*, 7th Edition, 1st Printing, page 59.

Delmar, *First Responder Handbook*, Fire Service Edition, page 76.

Mosby, *Emergency First Responder, Making the Difference*, 1st Edition, pages 106–108.

Jones and Bartlett, AAOS, *First Responder, Your First Response in Emergency Care*, 3rd Edition, page 52.

Answer: E

47. Reference: NFPA 1001, 4.3

Brady, *First Responder*, 7th Edition, 1st Printing, page 66.

Delmar, *First Responder Handbook*, Fire Service Edition, page 186.

Mosby, *Emergency First Responder, Making the Difference*, 1st Edition, page 63.

Jones and Bartlett, AAOS, *First Responder, Your First Response in Emergency Care*, 3rd Edition, page 54.

Answer: C

48. Reference: NFPA 1001, 4.3

Brady, *First Responder*, 7th Edition, 1st Printing, page 461.

Mosby, *Emergency First Responder, Making the Difference*, 1st Edition, pages 316–317 and 319.

Answer: B

49. Reference: NFPA 1001, 4.3

Brady, *First Responder*, 7th Edition, 1st Printing, page 463.

Delmar, *First Responder Handbook*, Fire Service Edition, page 302.

Jones and Bartlett, AAOS, *First Responder, Your First Response in Emergency Care*, 3rd Edition, pages 368–370.

Answer: D

50. Reference: NFPA 1001, 4.3

Brady, *First Responder*, 7th Edition, 1st Printing, page 463.

Delmar, *First Responder Handbook*, Fire Service Edition, page 301.

Mosby, *Emergency First Responder, Making the Difference*, 1st Edition, page 329.

Jones and Bartlett, AAOS, *First Responder, Your First Response in Emergency Care*, 3rd Edition, page 368.

Answer: C

51. Reference: NFPA 1001, 4.3
Brady, *First Responder*, 7th Edition, 1st Printing, page 464.
Answer: B

52. Reference: NFPA 1001, 4.3
Brady, *First Responder*, 7th Edition, 1st Printing, page 6.
Delmar, *First Responder Handbook*, Fire Service Edition, pages 57–58.
Mosby, *Emergency First Responder, Making the Difference*, 1st Edition, page 42.
Jones and Bartlett, AAOS, *First Responder, Your First Response in Emergency Care*, 3rd Edition, page 37.
Answer: B

53. Reference: NFPA 1001, 4.3
Brady, *First Responder*, 7th Edition, 1st Printing, page 8.
Delmar, *First Responder Handbook*, Fire Service Edition, pages 4–6.
Mosby, *Emergency First Responder, Making the Difference*, 1st Edition, pages 7, 9, and 13.
Jones and Bartlett, AAOS, *First Responder, Your First Response in Emergency Care*, 3rd Edition, page 4.
Answer: D

54. Reference: NFPA 1001, 4.3
Delmar, *First Responder Handbook*, Fire Service Edition, pages 13–15.
Mosby, *Emergency First Responder, Making the Difference*, 1st Edition, pages 4–5.
Jones and Bartlett, AAOS, *First Responder, Your First Response in Emergency Care*, 3rd Edition, page 8.
Answer: C

55. Reference: NFPA 1001, 4.3
Brady, *First Responder*, 7th Edition, 1st Printing, page 5.
Delmar, *First Responder Handbook*, Fire Service Edition, page 16.
Mosby, *Emergency First Responder, Making the Difference*, 1st Edition, page 7.
Answer: E

56. Reference: NFPA 1001, 4.3
Brady, *First Responder*, 7th Edition, 1st Printing, page 5.
Delmar, *First Responder Handbook*, Fire Service Edition, page 17.
Mosby, *Emergency First Responder, Making the Difference*, 1st Edition, page 8.
Jones and Bartlett, AAOS, *First Responder, Your First Response in Emergency Care*, 3rd Edition, page 11.
Answer: C

57. Reference: NFPA 1001, 4.3
Brady, *First Responder*, 7th Edition, 1st Printing, page 5.
Delmar, *First Responder Handbook*, Fire Service Edition, page 18.
Mosby, *Emergency First Responder, Making the Difference*, 1st Edition, page 11.
Jones and Bartlett, AAOS, *First Responder, Your First Response in Emergency Care*, 3rd Edition, page 15.
Answer: D

58. Reference: NFPA 1001, 4.3
Brady, *First Responder*, 7th Edition, 1st Printing, page 5.
Delmar, *First Responder Handbook*, Fire Service Edition, pages 18–19.
Mosby, *Emergency First Responder, Making the Difference*, 1st Edition, page 12.
Jones and Bartlett, AAOS, *First Responder, Your First Response in Emergency Care*, 3rd Edition, page 15.
Answer: A

59. Reference: NFPA 1001, 4.3
Brady, *First Responder*, 7th Edition, 1st Printing, page 29.
Delmar, *First Responder Handbook*, Fire Service Edition, page 67.
Mosby, *Emergency First Responder, Making the Difference*, 1st Edition, page 51.
Answer: D

60. Reference: NFPA 1001, 4.3
Brady, *First Responder*, 7th Edition, 1st Printing, pages 22 and 23.
Delmar, *First Responder Handbook*, Fire Service Edition, page 59.
Mosby, *Emergency First Responder, Making the Difference*, 1st Edition, page 12.
Jones and Bartlett, AAOS, *First Responder, Your First Response in Emergency Care*, 3rd Edition, pages 37 and 38.
Answer: A

61. Reference: NFPA 1001, 4.3
Brady, *First Responder*, 7th Edition, 1st Printing, page 22.
Delmar, *First Responder Handbook*, Fire Service Edition, page 59.
Mosby, *Emergency First Responder, Making the Difference*, 1st Edition, page 43.
Jones and Bartlett, AAOS, *First Responder, Your First Response in Emergency Care*, 3rd Edition, page 37.
Answer: B

62. Reference: NFPA 1001, 4.3
Brady, *First Responder*, 7th Edition, 1st Printing, page 23.
Delmar, *First Responder Handbook*, Fire Service Edition, page 59.
Mosby, *Emergency First Responder, Making the Difference*, 1st Edition, pages 43 and 44.
Jones and Bartlett, AAOS, *First Responder, Your First Response in Emergency Care*, 3rd Edition, page 38.
Answer: A

63. Reference: NFPA 1001, 4.3
Brady, *First Responder*, 7th Edition, 1st Printing, page 21.
Delmar, *First Responder Handbook*, Fire Service Edition, page 59.
Mosby, *Emergency First Responder, Making the Difference*, 1st Edition, page 44.
Jones and Bartlett, AAOS, *First Responder, Your First Response in Emergency Care*, 3rd Edition, page 39.
Answer: D

64. Reference: NFPA 1001, 4.3
Brady, *First Responder*, 7th Edition, 1st Printing, pages 27 and 28.
Delmar, *First Responder Handbook*, Fire Service Edition, page 61.
Mosby, *Emergency First Responder, Making the Difference*, 1st Edition, page 12.
Jones and Bartlett, AAOS, *First Responder, Your First Response in Emergency Care*, 3rd Edition, page 40.
Answer: E

65. Reference: NFPA 1001, 4.3
Brady, *First Responder*, 7th Edition, 1st Printing, page 25.
Delmar, *First Responder Handbook*, Fire Service Edition, page 61.
Mosby, *Emergency First Responder, Making the Difference*, 1st Edition, page 48.
Jones and Bartlett, AAOS, *First Responder, Your First Response in Emergency Care*, 3rd Edition, page 41.
Answer: E

66. Reference: NFPA 1001, 4.3
Brady, *First Responder*, 7th Edition, 1st Printing, page 70.
Delmar, *First Responder Handbook*, Fire Service Edition, page 100.
Mosby, *Emergency First Responder, Making the Difference*, 1st Edition, page 85.
Jones and Bartlett, AAOS, *First Responder, Your First Response in Emergency Care*, 3rd Edition, page 69.
Answer: B

67. Reference: NFPA 1001, 4.3
Brady, *First Responder*, 7th Edition, 1st Printing, page 70.
Delmar, *First Responder Handbook*, Fire Service Edition, page 100.
Mosby, *Emergency First Responder, Making the Difference*, 1st Edition, page 84.
Jones and Bartlett, AAOS, *First Responder, Your First Response in Emergency Care*, 3rd Edition, page 69.
Answer: A

68. Reference: NFPA 1001, 4.3
Brady, *First Responder*, 7th Edition, 1st Printing, page 70.
Delmar, *First Responder Handbook*, Fire Service Edition, pages 101 and 102.
Mosby, *Emergency First Responder, Making the Difference*, 1st Edition, page 85.
Jones and Bartlett, AAOS, *First Responder, Your First Response in Emergency Care*, 3rd Edition, page 69.
Answer: C

69. Reference: NFPA 1001, 4.3
Brady, *First Responder*, 7th Edition, 1st Printing, pages 83–85.
Delmar, *First Responder Handbook*, Fire Service Edition, page 118.
Mosby, *Emergency First Responder, Making the Difference*, 1st Edition, pages 97 and 98.
Jones and Bartlett, AAOS, *First Responder, Your First Response in Emergency Care*, 3rd Edition, pages 81–83.
Answer: E

70. Reference: NFPA 1001, 4.3
Brady, *First Responder*, 7th Edition, 1st Printing, page 80.
Delmar, *First Responder Handbook*, Fire Service Edition, page 103.
Mosby, *Emergency First Responder, Making the Difference*, 1st Edition, page 93.
Answer: A

71. Reference: NFPA 1001, 4.3
Brady, *First Responder*, 7th Edition, 1st Printing, pages 71–75.
Delmar, *First Responder Handbook*, Fire Service Edition, page 104.
Mosby, *Emergency First Responder, Making the Difference*, 1st Edition, page 87.
Answer: C

72. Reference: NFPA 1001, 4.3
Brady, *First Responder*, 7th Edition, 1st Printing, pages 246 and 247.
Delmar, *First Responder Handbook*, Fire Service Edition, page 221.
Mosby, *Emergency First Responder, Making the Difference*, 1st Edition, page 217.
Jones and Bartlett, AAOS, *First Responder, Your First Response in Emergency Care*, 3rd Edition, pages 204 and 462.
Answer: C

73. Reference: NFPA 1001, 4.3
Delmar, *First Responder Handbook*, Fire Service Edition, page 188.
Mosby, *Emergency First Responder, Making the Difference*, 1st Edition, page 213.
Jones and Bartlett, AAOS, *First Responder, Your First Response in Emergency Care*, 3rd Edition, page 211.
Answer: A

74. Reference: NFPA 1001, 4.3
Brady, *First Responder*, 7th Edition, 1st Printing, page 266.
Delmar, *First Responder Handbook*, Fire Service Edition, pages 222–223.
Mosby, *Emergency First Responder, Making the Difference*, 1st Edition, page 221.
Jones and Bartlett, AAOS, *First Responder, Your First Response in Emergency Care*, 3rd Edition, page 209.
Answer: B

75. Reference: NFPA 1001, 4.3
Brady, *First Responder*, 7th Edition, 1st Printing, page 269.
Delmar, *First Responder Handbook*, Fire Service Edition, pages 223–224.
Mosby, *Emergency First Responder, Making the Difference*, 1st Edition, page 220.
Jones and Bartlett, AAOS, *First Responder, Your First Response in Emergency Care*, 3rd Edition, page 208.
Answer: A

76. Reference: NFPA 1001, 4.3
Brady, *First Responder*, 7th Edition, 1st Printing, page 269.
Delmar, *First Responder Handbook*, Fire Service Edition, page 224.
Mosby, *Emergency First Responder, Making the Difference*, 1st Edition, page 220.
Jones and Bartlett, AAOS, *First Responder, Your First Response in Emergency Care*, 3rd Edition, page 209.
Answer: A

77. Reference: NFPA 1001, 4.3
Brady, *First Responder*, 7th Edition, 1st Printing, pages 261 and 262.
Delmar, *First Responder Handbook*, Fire Service Edition, pages 197–198.
Mosby, *Emergency First Responder, Making the Difference*, 1st Edition, page 226.
Jones and Bartlett, AAOS, First *Responder, Your First Response in Emergency Care*, 3rd Edition, page 258.
Answer: E

78. Reference: NFPA 1001, 4.3
Brady, *First Responder*, 7th Edition, 1st Printing, page 261.
Delmar, *First Responder Handbook*, Fire Service Edition, page 197.
Mosby, *Emergency First Responder, Making the Difference*, 1st Edition, page 224.
Jones and Bartlett, AAOS, *First Responder, Your First Response in Emergency Care*, 3rd Edition, page 222.
Answer: B

79. Reference: NFPA 1001, 4.3
Brady, *First Responder*, 7th Edition, 1st Printing, pages 265 and 266.
Delmar, *First Responder Handbook*, Fire Service Edition, pages 224–225.
Mosby, *Emergency First Responder, Making the Difference*, 1st Edition, pages 223 and 224.
Jones and Bartlett, AAOS, *First Responder, Your First Response in Emergency Care*, 3rd Edition, page 207.
Answer: C

80. Reference: NFPA 1001, 4.3
Brady, *First Responder*, 7th Edition, 1st Printing, page 528.
Delmar, *First Responder Handbook*, Fire Service Edition, pages 160, 327, and 340.
Mosby, *Emergency First Responder, Making the Difference*, 1st Edition, pages 166 and 351.
Jones and Bartlett, AAOS, *First Responder, Your First Response in Emergency Care*, 3rd Edition, page 400.
Answer: D

81. Reference: NFPA 1001, 4.3
Brady, *First Responder*, 7th Edition, 1st Printing, page 418.
Delmar, *First Responder Handbook*, Fire Service Edition, page 284.
Mosby, *Emergency First Responder, Making the Difference*, 1st Edition, pages 275 and 287.
Jones and Bartlett, AAOS, *First Responder, Your First Response in Emergency Care*, 3rd Edition, pages 311 and 313.
Answer: B

82. Reference: NFPA 1001, 4.3
Brady, *First Responder*, 7th Edition, 1st Printing, page 397.
Delmar, *First Responder Handbook*, Fire Service Edition, pages 285–286.
Mosby, *Emergency First Responder, Making the Difference*, 1st Edition, page 291, Box 11-6.
Jones and Bartlett, AAOS, *First Responder, Your First Response in Emergency Care*, 3rd Edition, page 310.
Answer: D

83. Reference: NFPA 1001, 4.3

Brady, *First Responder*, 7th Edition, 1st Printing, page 396.

Jones and Bartlett, AAOS, *First Responder, Your First Response in Emergency Care*, 3rd Edition, page 267.

Answer: D

84. Reference: NFPA 1001, 4.3

Brady, *First Responder*, 7th Edition, 1st Printing, page 391.

Mosby, *Emergency First Responder, Making the Difference*, 1st Edition, page 286.

Answer: C

85. Reference: NFPA 1001, 4.3

Brady, *First Responder*, 7th Edition, 1st Printing, page 394.

Delmar, *First Responder Handbook*, Fire Service Edition, page 86.

Mosby, *Emergency First Responder, Making the Difference*, 1st Edition, page 67.

Jones and Bartlett, AAOS, *First Responder, Your First Response in Emergency Care*, 3rd Edition, page 231.

Answer: A

86. Reference: NFPA 1001, 4.3

Brady, *First Responder*, 7th Edition, 1st Printing, page 380.

Mosby, *Emergency First Responder, Making the Difference*, 1st Edition, page 273.

Jones and Bartlett, AAOS, *First Responder, Your First Response in Emergency Care*, 3rd Edition, page 303.

Answer: C

87. Reference: NFPA 1001, 4.3

Brady, *First Responder*, 7th Edition, 1st Printing, page 370.

Mosby, *Emergency First Responder, Making the Difference*, 1st Edition, pages 269 and 270-271.

Answer: A

88. Reference: NFPA 1001, 4.3

Brady, *First Responder*, 7th Edition, 1st Printing, page 386.

Mosby, *Emergency First Responder, Making the Difference*, 1st Edition, pages 269 and 270–271.

Jones and Bartlett, AAOS, *First Responder, Your First Response in Emergency Care*, 3rd Edition, pages 292 and 295.

Answer: D

89. Reference: NFPA 1001, 4.3

Brady, *First Responder*, 7th Edition, 1st Printing, page 138.

Mosby, *Emergency First Responder, Making the Difference*, 1st Edition, pages 143–145.

Jones and Bartlett, AAOS, *First Responder, Your First Response in Emergency Care*, 3rd Edition, page 148.

Answer: A

90. Reference: NFPA 1001, 4.3

Brady, *First Responder*, 7th Edition, 1st Printing, page 138.

Mosby, *Emergency First Responder, Making the Difference*, 1st Edition, page 151.

Jones and Bartlett, AAOS, *First Responder, Your First Response in Emergency Care*, 3rd Edition, page 148.

Answer: D

91. Reference: NFPA 1001, 4.3

Brady, *First Responder*, 7th Edition, 1st Printing, page 138.

Mosby, *Emergency First Responder, Making the Difference*, 1st Edition, pages 140 and 142.

Jones and Bartlett, AAOS, *First Responder, Your First Response in Emergency Care*, 3rd Edition, pages 146 and 148.

Answer: C

92. Reference: NFPA 1001, 4.3

Brady, *First Responder*, 7th Edition, 1st Printing, page 141.

Mosby, *Emergency First Responder, Making the Difference*, 1st Edition, page 140.

Jones and Bartlett, AAOS, *First Responder, Your First Response in Emergency Care*, 3rd Edition, page 147.

Answer: C

93. Reference: NFPA 1001, 4.3

Brady, *First Responder*, 7th Edition, 1st Printing, page 138.

Delmar, *First Responder Handbook*, Fire Service Edition, page 160.

Mosby, *Emergency First Responder, Making the Difference*, 1st Edition, page 142.

Jones and Bartlett, AAOS, *First Responder, Your First Response in Emergency Care*, 3rd Edition, page 148.

Answer: C

94. Reference: NFPA 1001, 4.3

Brady, *First Responder*, 7th Edition, 1st Printing, page 153.

Mosby, *Emergency First Responder, Making the Difference*, 1st Edition, page 142.

Jones and Bartlett, AAOS, *First Responder, Your First Response in Emergency Care*, 3rd Edition, page 102.

Answer: B

95. Reference: NFPA 1001, 4.3

Brady, *First Responder*, 7th Edition, 1st Printing, page 48.

Delmar, *First Responder Handbook*, Fire Service Edition, pages 157 and 335.

Mosby, *Emergency First Responder, Making the Difference*, 1st Edition, pages 139–144.

Jones and Bartlett, AAOS, *First Responder, Your First Response in Emergency Care*, 3rd Edition, pages 386–387.

Answer: C

96. Reference: NFPA 1001, 4.3

Brady, *First Responder*, 7th Edition, 1st Printing, page 38.

Mosby, *Emergency First Responder, Making the Difference*, 1st Edition, page 48.

Jones and Bartlett, AAOS, *First Responder, Your First Response in Emergency Care*, 3rd Edition, page 42.

Answer: A

97. Reference: NFPA 1001, 4.3

Brady, *First Responder*, 7th Edition, 1st Printing, page 39.

Delmar, *First Responder Handbook*, Fire Service Edition, page 26.

Mosby, *Emergency First Responder, Making the Difference*, 1st Edition, pages 24–25.

Jones and Bartlett, AAOS, *First Responder, Your First Response in Emergency Care*, 3rd Edition, page 24.

Answer: C

98. Reference: NFPA 1001, 4.3
Brady, *First Responder*, 7th Edition, 1st Printing, page 39.
Delmar, *First Responder Handbook*, Fire Service Edition, page 26.
Mosby, *Emergency First Responder, Making the Difference*, 1st Edition, page 24.
Jones and Bartlett, AAOS, *First Responder, Your First Response in Emergency Care*, 3rd Edition, page 22.
Answer: E

99. Reference: NFPA 1001, 4.3
Brady, *First Responder*, 7th Edition, 1st Printing, page 39.
Delmar, *First Responder Handbook*, Fire Service Edition, page 30.
Mosby, *Emergency First Responder, Making the Difference*, 1st Edition, page 23.
Jones and Bartlett, AAOS, *First Responder, Your First Response in Emergency Care*, 3rd Edition, page 21.
Answer: C

100. Reference: NFPA 1001, 4.3
Brady, *First Responder*, 7th Edition, 1st Printing, page 39.
Delmar, *First Responder Handbook*, Fire Service Edition, page 30.
Mosby, *Emergency First Responder, Making the Difference*, 1st Edition, page 23.
Jones and Bartlett, AAOS, *First Responder, Your First Response in Emergency Care*, 3rd Edition, page 21.
Answer: B

Don't forget to enter the information on your Personal Progress Plotter and answer the Yes and No question at the end of the Examination. This step is extremely important for the successful completion of the Systematic Approach to Examination Preparation!

Examination I-2 Answer Key

Directions

Follow these steps carefully for completing the feedback part of SAEP:

1. After calculating your score, look up the answers for the examination items you missed as well as those on which you guessed, even if you guessed correctly. If you are guessing, it means the answer is not perfectly clear. In this process, we are committed to making you as knowledgeable as possible.

2. Enter the number of missed and guessed examination items in the blanks on your Personal Progress Plotter.

3. Highlight the answer in the reference materials. Read the paragraph preceding and the paragraph following the one in which the correct answer is located. Enter the paragraph number and page number next to the guessed or missed examination item on your examination. Count any part of a paragraph at the beginning of the page as one paragraph until you reach the paragraph containing your highlighted answer. This step will help you locate and review your missed and guessed examination items later in the process. It is essential to learning the material in context and by association. These learning techniques (context/association) are the very backbone of the SAEP approach.

4. Once you have completed the feedback part, you may proceed to the next examination.

1. Reference: NFPA 1001, 4.3

   Brady, *First Responder*, 7th Edition, 1st Printing, page 511.

   Delmar, *First Responder Handbook*, Fire Service Edition, page 332.

   Mosby, *Emergency First Responder, Making the Difference*, 1st Edition, page 347.

   Jones and Bartlett, AAOS, *First Responder, Your First Response in Emergency Care*, 3rd Edition, page 385.

   Answer: C

2. Reference: NFPA 1001, 4.3

   Brady, *First Responder*, 7th Edition, 1st Printing, pages 516–517.

   Delmar, *First Responder Handbook*, Fire Service Edition, page 335.

   Mosby, *Emergency First Responder, Making the Difference*, 1st Edition, pages 349–351.

   Jones and Bartlett, AAOS, *First Responder, Your First Response in Emergency Care*, 3rd Edition, pages 398–399.

   Answer: B

3. Reference: NFPA 1001, 4.3

   Brady, *First Responder*, 7th Edition, 1st Printing, page 521.

   Delmar, *First Responder Handbook*, Fire Service Edition, page 331.

   Mosby, *Emergency First Responder, Making the Difference*, 1st Edition, page 345.

   Jones and Bartlett, AAOS, *First Responder, Your First Response in Emergency Care*, 3rd Edition, page 385.

   Answer: D

4. Reference: NFPA 1001, 4.3
Brady, *First Responder*, 7th Edition, 1st Printing, page 521.
Delmar, *First Responder Handbook*, Fire Service Edition, page 330.
Mosby, *Emergency First Responder, Making the Difference*, 1st Edition, page 346.
Jones and Bartlett, AAOS, *First Responder, Your First Response in Emergency Care*, 3rd Edition, page 383.
Answer: A

5. Reference: NFPA 1001, 4.3
Brady, *First Responder*, 7th Edition, 1st Printing, page 552.
Delmar, *First Responder Handbook*, Fire Service Edition, page 151.
Jones and Bartlett, AAOS, *First Responder, Your First Response in Emergency Care*, 3rd Edition, page 442.
Answer: E

6. Reference: NFPA 1001, 4.3
Brady, *First Responder*, 7th Edition, 1st Printing, pages 96 and 132.
Delmar, *First Responder Handbook*, Fire Service Edition, page 124.
Mosby, *Emergency First Responder, Making the Difference*, 1st Edition, page 106.
Answer: D

7. Reference: NFPA 1001, 4.3
Brady, *First Responder*, 7th Edition, 1st Printing, page 97.
Answer: B

8. Reference: NFPA 1001, 4.3
Brady, *First Responder*, 7th Edition, 1st Printing, page 96.
Delmar, *First Responder Handbook*, Fire Service Edition, page 129.
Mosby, *Emergency First Responder, Making the Difference*, 1st Edition, page 60.
Jones and Bartlett, AAOS, *First Responder, Your First Response in Emergency Care*, 3rd Edition, page 105.
Answer: B

9. Reference: NFPA 1001, 4.3
Brady, *First Responder*, 7th Edition, 1st Printing, page 96.
Delmar, *First Responder Handbook*, Fire Service Edition, page 130.
Answer: B

10. Reference: NFPA 1001, 4.3
Brady, *First Responder*, 7th Edition, 1st Printing, pages 98 and 99.
Delmar, *First Responder Handbook*, Fire Service Edition, page 127.
Mosby, *Emergency First Responder, Making the Difference*, 1st Edition, page 108.
Answer: B

11. Reference: NFPA 1001, 4.3
Brady, *First Responder*, 7th Edition, 1st Printing, page 98.
Delmar, *First Responder Handbook*, Fire Service Edition, page 127.
Mosby, *Emergency First Responder, Making the Difference*, 1st Edition, page 108.
Jones and Bartlett, AAOS, *First Responder, Your First Response in Emergency Care*, 3rd Edition, page 52.
Answer: D

12. Reference: NFPA 1001, 4.3
Brady, *First Responder*, 7th Edition, 1st Printing, page 99.
Delmar, *First Responder Handbook*, Fire Service Edition, page 127.
Answer: B

13. Reference: NFPA 1001, 4.3
Brady, *First Responder*, 7th Edition, 1st Printing, pages 316–317.
Delmar, *First Responder Handbook*, Fire Service Edition, pages 240–241.
Mosby, *Emergency First Responder, Making the Difference*, 1st Edition, pages 247–248.
Jones and Bartlett, AAOS, *First Responder, Your First Response in Emergency Care*, 3rd Edition, page 267.
Answer: C

14. Reference: NFPA 1001, 4.3
Brady, *First Responder*, 7th Edition, 1st Printing, page 341.
Delmar, *First Responder Handbook*, Fire Service Edition, page 244.
Mosby, *Emergency First Responder, Making the Difference*, 1st Edition, page 253.
Jones and Bartlett, AAOS, *First Responder, Your First Response in Emergency Care*, 3rd Edition, page 278.
Answer: C

15. Reference: NFPA 1001, 4.3
Brady, *First Responder*, 7th Edition, 1st Printing, page 287.
Delmar, *First Responder Handbook*, Fire Service Edition, page 235.
Mosby, *Emergency First Responder, Making the Difference*, 1st Edition, page 239.
Jones and Bartlett, AAOS, *First Responder, Your First Response in Emergency Care*, 3rd Edition, page 264.
Answer: D

16. Reference: NFPA 1001, 4.3
Brady, *First Responder*, 7th Edition, 1st Printing, page 286.
Delmar, *First Responder Handbook*, Fire Service Edition, page 185.
Mosby, *Emergency First Responder, Making the Difference*, 1st Edition, page 242.
Answer: B

17. Reference: NFPA 1001, 4.3
Brady, *First Responder*, 7th Edition, 1st Printing, page 309.
Delmar, *First Responder Handbook*, Fire Service Edition, pages 198–199.
Mosby, *Emergency First Responder, Making the Difference*, 1st Edition, page 244.
Jones and Bartlett, AAOS, *First Responder, Your First Response in Emergency Care*, 3rd Edition, page 259.
Answer: A

18. Reference: NFPA 1001, 4.3
Brady, *First Responder*, 7th Edition, 1st Printing, page 308.
Delmar, *First Responder Handbook*, Fire Service Edition, page 196.
Mosby, *Emergency First Responder, Making the Difference*, 1st Edition, page 242.
Jones and Bartlett, AAOS, *First Responder, Your First Response in Emergency Care*, 3rd Edition, page 258.
Answer: E

19. Reference: NFPA 1001, 4.3
Brady, *First Responder*, 7th Edition, 1st Printing, pages 284–285.
Delmar, *First Responder Handbook*, Fire Service Edition, page 187.
Mosby, *Emergency First Responder, Making the Difference*, 1st Edition, pages 63 and 64.
Jones and Bartlett, AAOS, *First Responder, Your First Response in Emergency Care*, 3rd Edition, page 55.
Answer: A

20. Reference: NFPA 1001, 4.3
Brady, *First Responder*, 7th Edition, 1st Printing, page 436.
Delmar, *First Responder Handbook*, Fire Service Edition, page 319.
Mosby, *Emergency First Responder, Making the Difference*, 1st Edition, pages 303 and 304.
Jones and Bartlett, AAOS, *First Responder, Your First Response in Emergency Care*, 3rd Edition, page 339.
Answer: C

21. Reference: NFPA 1001, 4.3
Brady, *First Responder*, 7th Edition, 1st Printing, page 443.
Mosby, *Emergency First Responder, Making the Difference*, 1st Edition, page 298.
Jones and Bartlett, AAOS, *First Responder, Your First Response in Emergency Care*, 3rd Edition, page 341.
Answer: B

22. Reference: NFPA 1001, 4.3
Brady, *First Responder*, 7th Edition, 1st Printing, page 446.
Mosby, *Emergency First Responder, Making the Difference*, 1st Edition, page 307.
Jones and Bartlett, AAOS, *First Responder, Your First Response in Emergency Care*, 3rd Edition, page 343.
Answer: D

23. Reference: NFPA 1001, 4.3
Brady, *First Responder*, 7th Edition, 1st Printing, page 446.
Delmar, *First Responder Handbook*, Fire Service Edition, page 311.
Answer: A

24. Reference: NFPA 1001, 4.3
Brady, *First Responder*, 7th Edition, 1st Printing, pages 446 and 447.
Jones and Bartlett, AAOS, *First Responder, Your First Response in Emergency Care*, 3rd Edition, page 341.
Answer: D

25. Reference: NFPA 1001, 4.3
Brady, *First Responder*, 7th Edition, 1st Printing, page 215.
Mosby, *Emergency First Responder, Making the Difference*, 1st Edition, page 187.
Jones and Bartlett, AAOS, *First Responder, Your First Response in Emergency Care*, 3rd Edition, page 189.
Answer: B

26. Reference: NFPA 1001, 4.3
Brady, *First Responder*, 7th Edition, 1st Printing, page 195.
Mosby, *Emergency First Responder, Making the Difference*, 1st Edition, page 186.
Jones and Bartlett, AAOS, *First Responder, Your First Response in Emergency Care*, 3rd Edition, page 183.
Answer: B

27. Reference: NFPA 1001, 4.3
Brady, *First Responder*, 7th Edition, 1st Printing, pages 194 and 195.
Mosby, *Emergency First Responder, Making the Difference*, 1st Edition, page 186.
Jones and Bartlett, AAOS, *First Responder, Your First Response in Emergency Care*, 3rd Edition, page 183.
Answer: D

28. Reference: NFPA 1001, 4.3
Brady, *First Responder*, 7th Edition, 1st Printing, pages 194 and 195.
Mosby, *Emergency First Responder, Making the Difference*, 1st Edition, page 186.
Jones and Bartlett, AAOS, *First Responder, Your First Response in Emergency Care*, 3rd Edition, page 183.
Answer: C

29. Reference: NFPA 1001, 4.3
Brady, *First Responder*, 7th Edition, 1st Printing, page 212.
Mosby, *Emergency First Responder, Making the Difference*, 1st Edition, page 192.
Jones and Bartlett, AAOS, *First Responder, Your First Response in Emergency Care*, 3rd Edition, page 191.
Answer: C

30. Reference: NFPA 1001, 4.3
Brady, *First Responder*, 7th Edition, 1st Printing, page 212.
Delmar, *First Responder Handbook*, Fire Service Edition, page 167.
Mosby, *Emergency First Responder, Making the Difference*, 1st Edition, page 192.
Jones and Bartlett, AAOS, *First Responder, Your First Response in Emergency Care*, 3rd Edition, page 189.
Answer: A

31. Reference: NFPA 1001, 4.3
Brady, *First Responder*, 7th Edition, 1st Printing, page 212.
Mosby, *Emergency First Responder, Making the Difference*, 1st Edition, page 184.
Jones and Bartlett, AAOS, *First Responder, Your First Response in Emergency Care*, 3rd Edition, page 190.
Answer: D

32. Reference: NFPA 1001, 4.3
Brady, *First Responder*, 7th Edition, 1st Printing, page 213.
Delmar, *First Responder Handbook*, Fire Service Edition, page 142.
Mosby, *Emergency First Responder, Making the Difference*, 1st Edition, page 185.
Jones and Bartlett, AAOS, *First Responder, Your First Response in Emergency Care*, 3rd Edition, pages 189 and 191.
Answer: C

33. Reference: NFPA 1001, 4.3

Brady, *First Responder*, 7th Edition, 1st Printing, pages 213 and 217.

Delmar, *First Responder Handbook*, Fire Service Edition, page 319.

Mosby, *Emergency First Responder, Making the Difference*, 1st Edition, page 304.

Jones and Bartlett, AAOS, *First Responder, Your First Response in Emergency Care*, 3rd Edition, page 339.

Answer: A

34. Reference: NFPA 1001, 4.3

Delmar, *First Responder Handbook*, Fire Service Edition, page 79.

Mosby, *Emergency First Responder, Making the Difference*, 1st Edition, pages 69 and 72.

Jones and Bartlett, AAOS, *First Responder, Your First Response in Emergency Care*, 3rd Edition, page 460.

Answer: C

35. Reference: NFPA 1001, 4.3

Delmar, *First Responder Handbook*, Fire Service Edition, pages 79–82.

Mosby, *Emergency First Responder, Making the Difference*, 1st Edition, page 72.

Jones and Bartlett, AAOS, *First Responder, Your First Response in Emergency Care*, 3rd Edition, page 60.

Answer: C

36. Reference: NFPA 1001, 4.3

Delmar, *First Responder Handbook*, Fire Service Edition, page 82.

Mosby, *Emergency First Responder, Making the Difference*, 1st Edition, page 268.

Answer: B

37. Reference: NFPA 1001, 4.3

Brady, *First Responder*, 7th Edition, 1st Printing, page 62.

Answer: D

38. Reference: NFPA 1001, 4.3

Brady, *First Responder*, 7th Edition, 1st Printing, page 62.

Delmar, *First Responder Handbook*, Fire Service Edition, page 76.

Mosby, *Emergency First Responder, Making the Difference*, 1st Edition, pages 69 and 70.

Jones and Bartlett, AAOS, *First Responder, Your First Response in Emergency Care*, 3rd Edition, pages 58 and 59.

Answer: B

39. Reference: NFPA 1001, 4.3

Brady, *First Responder*, 7th Edition, 1st Printing, page 61.

Delmar, *First Responder Handbook*, Fire Service Edition, pages 87–88.

Mosby, *Emergency First Responder, Making the Difference*, 1st Edition, page 72.

Jones and Bartlett, AAOS, *First Responder, Your First Response in Emergency Care*, 3rd Edition, pages 62–63.

Answer: C

40. Reference: NFPA 1001, 4.3

Brady, *First Responder*, 7th Edition, 1st Printing, page 471.

Mosby, *Emergency First Responder, Making the Difference*, 1st Edition, page 370.

Jones and Bartlett, AAOS, *First Responder, Your First Response in Emergency Care*, 3rd Edition, pages 362–363.

Answer: C

41. Reference: NFPA 1001, 4.3

Brady, *First Responder*, 7th Edition, 1st Printing, pages 477 and 478.

Delmar, *First Responder Handbook*, Fire Service Edition, page 300.

Mosby, *Emergency First Responder, Making the Difference*, 1st Edition, page 328.

Jones and Bartlett, AAOS, *First Responder, Your First Response in Emergency Care*, 3rd Edition, page 367.

Answer: A

42. Reference: NFPA 1001, 4.3

Brady, *First Responder*, 7th Edition, 1st Printing, page 480.

Delmar, *First Responder Handbook*, Fire Service Edition, page 299.

Mosby, *Emergency First Responder, Making the Difference*, 1st Edition, page 326.

Jones and Bartlett, AAOS, *First Responder, Your First Response in Emergency Care*, 3rd Edition, page 365.

Answer: A

43. Reference: NFPA 1001, 4.3

Brady, *First Responder*, 7th Edition, 1st Printing, page 5.

Delmar, *First Responder Handbook*, Fire Service Edition, page 18.

Mosby, *Emergency First Responder, Making the Difference*, 1st Edition, page 4.

Answer: E

44. Reference: NFPA 1001, 4.3

Brady, *First Responder*, 7th Edition, 1st Printing, page 7.

Delmar, *First Responder Handbook*, Fire Service Edition, page 16.

Mosby, *Emergency First Responder, Making the Difference*, 1st Edition, page 8.

Jones and Bartlett, AAOS, *First Responder, Your First Response in Emergency Care*, 3rd Edition, page 11.

Answer: E

45. Reference: NFPA 1001, 4.3

Brady, *First Responder*, 7th Edition, 1st Printing, page 5.

Delmar, *First Responder Handbook*, Fire Service Edition, pages 18–19.

Mosby, *Emergency First Responder, Making the Difference*, 1st Edition, page 12.

Jones and Bartlett, AAOS, *First Responder, Your First Response in Emergency Care*, 3rd Edition, page 15.

Answer: A

46. Reference: NFPA 1001, 4.3
Brady, *First Responder*, 7th Edition, 1st Printing, page 3.
Delmar, *First Responder Handbook*, Fire Service Edition, page 5.
Mosby, *Emergency First Responder, Making the Difference*, 1st Edition, pages 2, 6, and 181.
Jones and Bartlett, AAOS, *First Responder, Your First Response in Emergency Care*, 3rd Edition, page 8.
Answer: D

47. Reference: NFPA 1001, 4.3
Brady, *First Responder*, 7th Edition, 1st Printing, page 3.
Delmar, *First Responder Handbook*, Fire Service Edition, page 3.
Mosby, *Emergency First Responder, Making the Difference*, 1st Edition, page 7.
Jones and Bartlett, AAOS, *First Responder, Your First Response in Emergency Care*, 3rd Edition, page 4.
Answer: B

48. Reference: NFPA 1001, 4.3
Brady, *First Responder*, 7th Edition, 1st Printing, page 25.
Delmar, *First Responder Handbook*, Fire Service Edition, page 61.
Mosby, *Emergency First Responder, Making the Difference*, 1st Edition, pages 48–49.
Jones and Bartlett, AAOS, *First Responder, Your First Response in Emergency Care*, 3rd Edition, pages 40 and 41.
Answer: C

49. Reference: NFPA 1001, 4.3
Brady, *First Responder*, 7th Edition, 1st Printing, page 21.
Delmar, *First Responder Handbook*, Fire Service Edition, page 61.
Mosby, *Emergency First Responder, Making the Difference*, 1st Edition, page 47.
Answer: D

50. Reference: NFPA 1001, 4.3
Brady, *First Responder*, 7th Edition, 1st Printing, page 23.
Delmar, *First Responder Handbook*, Fire Service Edition, page 62.
Mosby, *Emergency First Responder, Making the Difference*, 1st Edition, page 46.
Jones and Bartlett, AAOS, *First Responder, Your First Response in Emergency Care*, 3rd Edition, pages 39 and 40.
Answer: A

51. Reference: NFPA 1001, 4.3
Brady, *First Responder*, 7th Edition, 1st Printing, pages 23 and 24.
Delmar, *First Responder Handbook*, Fire Service Edition, pages 62–63.
Mosby, *Emergency First Responder, Making the Difference*, 1st Edition, pages 46–47.
Jones and Bartlett, AAOS, *First Responder, Your First Response in Emergency Care*, 3rd Edition, pages 39 and 40.
Answer: B

52. Reference: NFPA 1001, 4.3
Brady, *First Responder*, 7th Edition, 1st Printing, page 23.
Delmar, *First Responder Handbook*, Fire Service Edition, pages 59–60.
Mosby, *Emergency First Responder, Making the Difference*, 1st Edition, page 45.
Jones and Bartlett, AAOS, *First Responder, Your First Response in Emergency Care*,
3rd Edition, page 38.
Answer: A

53. Reference: NFPA 1001, 4.3
Delmar, *First Responder Handbook*, Fire Service Edition, pages 98–102.
Mosby, *Emergency First Responder, Making the Difference*, 1st Edition, pages 84–85.
Jones and Bartlett, AAOS, *First Responder, Your First Response in Emergency Care*,
3rd Edition, pages 69–70.
Answer: D

54. Reference: NFPA 1001, 4.3
Brady, *First Responder*, 7th Edition, 1st Printing, pages 70–72.
Delmar, *First Responder Handbook*, Fire Service Edition, page 103.
Mosby, *Emergency First Responder, Making the Difference*, 1st Edition, page 85.
Jones and Bartlett, AAOS, *First Responder, Your First Response in Emergency Care*,
3rd Edition, page 70.
Answer: B

55. Reference: NFPA 1001, 4.3
Brady, *First Responder*, 7th Edition, 1st Printing, page 69.
Delmar, *First Responder Handbook*, Fire Service Edition, page 100.
Mosby, *Emergency First Responder, Making the Difference*, 1st Edition, page 84.
Jones and Bartlett, AAOS, *First Responder, Your First Response in Emergency Care*,
3rd Edition, page 69.
Answer: C

56. Reference: NFPA 1001, 4.3
Brady, *First Responder*, 7th Edition, 1st Printing, page 71.
Delmar, *First Responder Handbook*, Fire Service Edition, page 103.
Mosby, *Emergency First Responder, Making the Difference*, 1st Edition, page 87.
Jones and Bartlett, AAOS, *First Responder, Your First Response in Emergency Care*,
3rd Edition, page 70.
Answer: A

57. Reference: NFPA 1001, 4.3
Brady, *First Responder*, 7th Edition, 1st Printing, page 71.
Delmar, *First Responder Handbook*, Fire Service Edition, page 103.
Mosby, *Emergency First Responder, Making the Difference*, 1st Edition, page 87.
Jones and Bartlett, AAOS, *First Responder, Your First Response in Emergency Care*,
3rd Edition, page 70.
Answer: B

58. Reference: NFPA 1001, 4.3
Delmar, *First Responder Handbook*, Fire Service Edition, page 222.
Mosby, *Emergency First Responder, Making the Difference*, 1st Edition, page 327.
Answer: E

59. Reference: NFPA 1001, 4.3

Brady, *First Responder*, 7th Edition, 1st Printing, page 250.

Mosby, *Emergency First Responder, Making the Difference*, 1st Edition, page 216.

Answer: A

60. Reference: NFPA 1001, 4.3

Brady, *First Responder*, 7th Edition, 1st Printing, page 247.

Mosby, *Emergency First Responder, Making the Difference*, 1st Edition, page 217.

Jones and Bartlett, AAOS, *First Responder, Your First Response in Emergency Care*, 3rd Edition, page 205.

Answer: D

61. Reference: NFPA 1001, 4.3

Brady, *First Responder*, 7th Edition, 1st Printing, pages 245–246.

Mosby, *Emergency First Responder, Making the Difference*, 1st Edition, page 218.

Jones and Bartlett, AAOS, *First Responder, Your First Response in Emergency Care*, 3rd Edition, page 214.

Answer: A

62. Reference: NFPA 1001, 4.3

Brady, *First Responder*, 7th Edition, 1st Printing, pages 244 and 245.

Mosby, *Emergency First Responder, Making the Difference*, 1st Edition, page 219.

Jones and Bartlett, AAOS, *First Responder, Your First Response in Emergency Care*, 3rd Edition, page 214.

Answer: C

63. Reference: NFPA 1001, 4.3

Brady, *First Responder*, 7th Edition, 1st Printing, page 239.

Delmar, *First Responder Handbook*, Fire Service Edition, pages 130–131.

Mosby, *Emergency First Responder, Making the Difference*, 1st Edition, pages 212–213 and 326.

Jones and Bartlett, AAOS, *First Responder, Your First Response in Emergency Care*, 3rd Edition, pages 210 and 360.

Answer: B

64. Reference: NFPA 1001, 4.3

Brady, *First Responder*, 7th Edition, 1st Printing, page 527.

Delmar, *First Responder Handbook*, Fire Service Edition, page 341.

Mosby, *Emergency First Responder, Making the Difference*, 1st Edition, page 343.

Jones and Bartlett, AAOS, *First Responder, Your First Response in Emergency Care*, 3rd Edition, page 406.

Answer: D

65. Reference: NFPA 1001, 4.3

Brady, *First Responder*, 7th Edition, 1st Printing, page 371.

Delmar, *First Responder Handbook*, Fire Service Edition, pages 263–264.

Mosby, *Emergency First Responder, Making the Difference*, 1st Edition, page 273.

Jones and Bartlett, AAOS, *First Responder, Your First Response in Emergency Care*, 3rd Edition, page 299.

Answer: D

66. Reference: NFPA 1001, 4.3
Brady, *First Responder*, 7th Edition, 1st Printing, page 365.
Delmar, *First Responder Handbook*, Fire Service Edition, page 262.
Mosby, *Emergency First Responder, Making the Difference*, 1st Edition, page 273.
Jones and Bartlett, AAOS, *First Responder, Your First Response in Emergency Care*, 3rd Edition, page 297.
Answer: B

67. Reference: NFPA 1001, 4.3
Brady, *First Responder*, 7th Edition, 1st Printing, page 362.
Delmar, *First Responder Handbook*, Fire Service Edition, pages 262–264.
Mosby, *Emergency First Responder, Making the Difference*, 1st Edition, page 270.
Jones and Bartlett, AAOS, *First Responder, Your First Response in Emergency Care*, 3rd Edition, page 295.
Answer: D

68. Reference: NFPA 1001, 4.3
Brady, *First Responder*, 7th Edition, 1st Printing, page 361.
Mosby, *Emergency First Responder, Making the Difference*, 1st Edition, pages 268–269.
Jones and Bartlett, AAOS, *First Responder, Your First Response in Emergency Care*, 3rd Edition, page 291.
Answer: A

69. Reference: NFPA 1001, 4.3
Brady, *First Responder*, 7th Edition, 1st Printing, page 370.
Answer: C

70. Reference: NFPA 1001, 4.3
Brady, *First Responder*, 7th Edition, 1st Printing, page 356.
Delmar, *First Responder Handbook*, Fire Service Edition, page 79.
Mosby, *Emergency First Responder, Making the Difference*, 1st Edition, page 269.
Jones and Bartlett, AAOS, *First Responder, Your First Response in Emergency Care*, 3rd Edition, page 286.
Answer: C

71. Reference: NFPA 1001, 4.3
Brady, *First Responder*, 7th Edition, 1st Printing, page 354.
Delmar, *First Responder Handbook*, Fire Service Edition, pages 76 and 79.
Mosby, *Emergency First Responder, Making the Difference*, 1st Edition, page 264.
Jones and Bartlett, AAOS, *First Responder, Your First Response in Emergency Care*, 3rd Edition, pages 286–287.
Answer: A

72. Reference: NFPA 1001, 4.3
Brady, *First Responder*, 7th Edition, 1st Printing, page 150.
Delmar, *First Responder Handbook*, Fire Service Edition, page 156.
Mosby, *Emergency First Responder, Making the Difference*, 1st Edition, page 185.
Answer: A

73. Reference: NFPA 1001, 4.3

Brady, *First Responder*, 7th Edition, 1st Printing, page 157.
Delmar, *First Responder Handbook*, Fire Service Edition, page 267.
Mosby, *Emergency First Responder, Making the Difference*, 1st Edition, page 166.
Jones and Bartlett, AAOS, *First Responder, Your First Response in Emergency Care*, 3rd Edition, page 153.
Answer: C

74. Reference: NFPA 1001, 4.3

Brady, *First Responder*, 7th Edition, 1st Printing, page 166.
Delmar, *First Responder Handbook*, Fire Service Edition, pages 175–177.
Mosby, *Emergency First Responder, Making the Difference*, 1st Edition, pages 163–167.
Jones and Bartlett, AAOS, *First Responder, Your First Response in Emergency Care*, 3rd Edition, pages 152–154.
Answer: B

75. Reference: NFPA 1001, 4.3

Brady, *First Responder*, 7th Edition, 1st Printing, page 160.
Delmar, *First Responder Handbook*, Fire Service Edition, page 159.
Mosby, *Emergency First Responder, Making the Difference*, 1st Edition, page 143, Table 7-2.
Jones and Bartlett, AAOS, *First Responder, Your First Response in Emergency Care*, 3rd Edition, page 158.
Answer: C

76. Reference: NFPA 1001, 4.3

Brady, *First Responder*, 7th Edition, 1st Printing, page 163.
Mosby, *Emergency First Responder, Making the Difference*, 1st Edition, page 145.
Answer: D

77. Reference: NFPA 1001, 4.3

Brady, *First Responder*, 7th Edition, 1st Printing, page 164.
Delmar, *First Responder Handbook*, Fire Service Edition, pages 179 and 180.
Mosby, *Emergency First Responder, Making the Difference*, 1st Edition, page 162.
Jones and Bartlett, AAOS, *First Responder, Your First Response in Emergency Care*, 3rd Edition, page 216.
Answer: B

78. Reference: NFPA 1001, 4.3

Brady, *First Responder*, 7th Edition, 1st Printing, page 164.
Answer: C

79. Reference: NFPA 1001, 4.3

Brady, *First Responder*, 7th Edition, 1st Printing, page 167.
Answer: D

80. Reference: NFPA 1001, 4.3

Brady, *First Responder*, 7th Edition, 1st Printing, page 171.
Answer: C

81. Reference: NFPA 1001, 4.3

Brady, *First Responder*, 7th Edition, 1st Printing, pages 154, 244, 256, and 596.

Delmar, *First Responder Handbook*, Fire Service Edition, page 161.

Mosby, *Emergency First Responder, Making the Difference*, 1st Edition, page 145.

Jones and Bartlett, AAOS, *First Responder, Your First Response in Emergency Care*, 3rd Edition, page 149.

Answer: C

82. Reference: NFPA 1001, 4.3

Brady, *First Responder*, 7th Edition, 1st Printing, page 178.

Delmar, *First Responder Handbook*, Fire Service Edition, page 180.

Mosby, *Emergency First Responder, Making the Difference*, 1st Edition, page 162.

Jones and Bartlett, AAOS, *First Responder, Your First Response in Emergency Care*, 3rd Edition, page 163.

Answer: C

83. Reference: NFPA 1001, 4.3

Brady, *First Responder*, 7th Edition, 1st Printing, page 165.

Delmar, *First Responder Handbook*, Fire Service Edition, page 179.

Mosby, *Emergency First Responder, Making the Difference*, 1st Edition, page 161, Table 7-9.

Jones and Bartlett, AAOS, *First Responder, Your First Response in Emergency Care*, 3rd Edition, page 162.

Answer: B

84. Reference: NFPA 1001, 4.3

Brady, *First Responder*, 7th Edition, 1st Printing, pages 399 and 542.

Delmar, *First Responder Handbook*, Fire Service Edition, page 178.

Mosby, *Emergency First Responder, Making the Difference*, 1st Edition, page 163.

Jones and Bartlett, AAOS, *First Responder, Your First Response in Emergency Care*, 3rd Edition, page 438.

Answer: C

85. Reference: NFPA 1001, 4.3

Delmar, *First Responder Handbook*, Fire Service Edition, page 162.

Mosby, *Emergency First Responder, Making the Difference*, 1st Edition, pages 145–146.

Jones and Bartlett, AAOS, *First Responder, Your First Response in Emergency Care*, 3rd Edition, page 149.

Answer: D

86. Reference: NFPA 1001, 4.3

Brady, *First Responder*, 7th Edition, 1st Printing, page 168.

Delmar, *First Responder Handbook*, Fire Service Edition, page 175.

Mosby, *Emergency First Responder, Making the Difference*, 1st Edition, pages 22 and 163.

Answer: E

87. Reference: NFPA 1001, 4.3

Brady, *First Responder*, 7th Edition, 1st Printing, page 170.

Delmar, *First Responder Handbook*, Fire Service Edition, page 164.

Mosby, *Emergency First Responder, Making the Difference*, 1st Edition, page 163.

Jones and Bartlett, AAOS, *First Responder, Your First Response in Emergency Care*, 3rd Edition, page 152.

Answer: B

88. Reference: NFPA 1001, 4.3

Delmar, *First Responder Handbook*, Fire Service Edition, pages 31–32.

Mosby, *Emergency First Responder, Making the Difference*, 1st Edition, page 26.

Jones and Bartlett, AAOS, *First Responder, Your First Response in Emergency Care*, 3rd Edition, page 371.

Answer: D

89. Reference: NFPA 1001, 4.3

Delmar, *First Responder Handbook*, Fire Service Edition, page 31.

Mosby, *Emergency First Responder, Making the Difference*, 1st Edition, page 25.

Jones and Bartlett, AAOS, *First Responder, Your First Response in Emergency Care*, 3rd Edition, pages 248–249.

Answer: A

90. Reference: NFPA 1001, 4.3

Brady, *First Responder*, 7th Edition, 1st Printing, page 41.

Delmar, *First Responder Handbook*, Fire Service Edition, page 32.

Mosby, *Emergency First Responder, Making the Difference*, 1st Edition, page 26, Box 2-3.

Jones and Bartlett, AAOS, *First Responder, Your First Response in Emergency Care*, 3rd Edition, page 25.

Answer: B

91. Reference: NFPA 1001, 4.3

Brady, *First Responder*, 7th Edition, 1st Printing, pages 36, 37, and 41.

Delmar, *First Responder Handbook*, Fire Service Edition, pages 31–33.

Mosby, *Emergency First Responder, Making the Difference*, 1st Edition, page 25.

Jones and Bartlett, AAOS, *First Responder, Your First Response in Emergency Care*, 3rd Edition, page 25.

Answer: E

92. Reference: NFPA 1001, 4.3

Brady, *First Responder*, 7th Edition, 1st Printing, pages 8 and 36–37.

Delmar, *First Responder Handbook*, Fire Service Edition, pages 24–49.

Mosby, *Emergency First Responder, Making the Difference*, 1st Edition, pages 24, 26, and 31.

Jones and Bartlett, AAOS, *First Responder, Your First Response in Emergency Care*, 3rd Edition, pages 25, 26, and 27.

Answer: B

93. Reference: NFPA 1001, 4.3

Brady, *First Responder*, 7th Edition, 1st Printing, page 43.

Delmar, *First Responder Handbook*, Fire Service Edition, page 42.

Answer: B

94. Reference: NFPA 1001, 4.3
Brady, *First Responder*, 7th Edition, 1st Printing, page 39.
Mosby, *Emergency First Responder, Making the Difference*, 1st Edition, page 24.
Jones and Bartlett, AAOS, *First Responder, Your First Response in Emergency Care*, 3rd Edition, page 242.
Answer: A

95. Reference: NFPA 1001, 4.3
Brady, *First Responder*, 7th Edition, 1st Printing, page 42.
Delmar, *First Responder Handbook*, Fire Service Edition, page 42.
Mosby, *Emergency First Responder, Making the Difference*, 1st Edition, page 26.
Jones and Bartlett, AAOS, *First Responder, Your First Response in Emergency Care*, 3rd Edition, page 26.
Answer: A

96. Reference: NFPA 1001, 4.3
Brady, *First Responder*, 7th Edition, 1st Printing, page 39.
Delmar, *First Responder Handbook*, Fire Service Edition, page 26.
Mosby, *Emergency First Responder, Making the Difference*, 1st Edition, page 24.
Jones and Bartlett, AAOS, *First Responder, Your First Response in Emergency Care*, 3rd Edition, page 22.
Answer: D

97. Reference: NFPA 1001, 4.3
Brady, *First Responder*, 7th Edition, 1st Printing, pages 44 and 191.
Delmar, *First Responder Handbook*, Fire Service Edition, pages 42–49.
Mosby, *Emergency First Responder, Making the Difference*, 1st Edition, pages 26 and 115.
Jones and Bartlett, AAOS, *First Responder, Your First Response in Emergency Care*, 3rd Edition, pages 26–27.
Answer: C

98. Reference: NFPA 1001, 4.3
Delmar, *First Responder Handbook*, Fire Service Edition, page 45.
Answer: D

99. Reference: NFPA 1001, 4.3
Brady, *First Responder*, 7th Edition, 1st Printing, page 47.
Delmar, *First Responder Handbook*, Fire Service Edition, pages 50–51.
Jones and Bartlett, AAOS, *First Responder, Your First Response in Emergency Care*, 3rd Edition, page 27.
Answer: D

100. Reference: NFPA 1001, 4.3
Delmar, *First Responder Handbook*, Fire Service Edition, page 44.
Jones and Bartlett, AAOS, *First Responder, Your First Response in Emergency Care*, 3rd Edition, page 26.
Answer: A

Don't forget to enter the information on your Personal Progress Plotter and answer the Yes and No question at the end of the Examination. This step is extremely important for the successful completion of the Systematic Approach to Examination Preparation!

Examination I-3 Answer Key

Directions
Follow these steps carefully for completing the feedback part of SAEP:

1. After calculating your score, look up the answers for the examination items you missed as well as those on which you guessed, even if you guessed correctly. If you are guessing, it means the answer is not perfectly clear. In this process, we are committed to making you as knowledgeable as possible.

2. Enter the number of missed and guessed examination items in the blanks on your Personal Progress Plotter.

3. Highlight the answer in the reference materials. Read the paragraph preceding and the paragraph following the one in which the correct answer is located. Enter the paragraph number and page number next to the guessed or missed examination item on your examination. Count any part of a paragraph at the beginning of the page as one paragraph until you reach the paragraph containing your highlighted answer. This step will help you locate and review your missed and guessed examination items later in the process. It is essential to learning the material in context and by association. These learning techniques (context/association) are the very backbone of the SAEP approach.

4. Congratulations! You have completed the examination and feedback steps of SAEP when you have highlighted your guessed and missed examination items for this examination.

Proceed to Phases II and III. Study the materials carefully in these important phases—they will help you polish your examination-taking skills. Approximately two to three days before you take your next examination, carefully read all of the highlighted information in the reference materials using the same techniques you applied during the feedback step. This will reinforce your learning and provide you with an added level of confidence going into the examination.

Someone once said to professional golfer Tom Watson after he won several tournament championships, "You are really lucky to have won those championships. You are really on a streak." Watson was reported to have replied, "Yes, there is some luck involved, but what I have really noticed is that the more I practice, the luckier I get." What Watson was saying is that good luck usually results from good preparation. This line of thinking certainly applies to learning the rules and hints of examination taking.

——————— **Rule 7** ———————

Good luck = good preparation.

1. Reference: NFPA 1001, 4.3
   Brady, *First Responder*, 7th Edition, 1st Printing, page 507.
   Answer: D

2. Reference: NFPA 1001, 4.3
   Brady, *First Responder*, 7th Edition, 1st Printing, pages 516–517.
   Delmar, *First Responder Handbook*, Fire Service Edition, page 335.
   Mosby, *Emergency First Responder, Making the Difference*, 1st Edition, pages 349–351.
   Jones and Bartlett, AAOS, *First Responder, Your First Response in Emergency Care*, 3rd Edition, pages 398–399.
   Answer: B

3. Reference: NFPA 1001, 4.3

Brady, *First Responder*, 7th Edition, 1st Printing, page 521.

Delmar, *First Responder Handbook*, Fire Service Edition, page 326.

Mosby, *Emergency First Responder, Making the Difference*, 1st Edition, page 345.

Jones and Bartlett, AAOS, *First Responder, Your First Response in Emergency Care*, 3rd Edition, page 383.

Answer: D

4. Reference: NFPA 1001, 4.3

Brady, *First Responder*, 7th Edition, 1st Printing, pages 98 and 99.

Delmar, *First Responder Handbook*, Fire Service Edition, page 125.

Mosby, *Emergency First Responder, Making the Difference*, 1st Edition, page 106.

Jones and Bartlett, AAOS, *First Responder, Your First Response in Emergency Care*, 3rd Edition, page 104.

Answer: C

5. Reference: NFPA 1001, 4.3

Brady, *First Responder*, 7th Edition, 1st Printing, pages 102 and 111.

Delmar, *First Responder Handbook*, Fire Service Edition, pages 131–132.

Mosby, *Emergency First Responder, Making the Difference*, 1st Edition, page 109.

Jones and Bartlett, AAOS, *First Responder, Your First Response in Emergency Care*, 3rd Edition, page 107.

Answer: B

6. Reference: NFPA 1001, 4.3

Brady, *First Responder*, 7th Edition, 1st Printing, page 121.

Delmar, *First Responder Handbook*, Fire Service Edition, page 138.

Mosby, *Emergency First Responder, Making the Difference*, 1st Edition, page 109.

Jones and Bartlett, AAOS, *First Responder, Your First Response in Emergency Care*, 3rd Edition, page 109.

Answer: C

7. Reference: NFPA 1001, 4.3

Brady, *First Responder*, 7th Edition, 1st Printing, page 97.

Answer: B

8. Reference: NFPA 1001, 4.3

Brady, *First Responder*, 7th Edition, 1st Printing, pages 98 and 99.

Delmar, *First Responder Handbook*, Fire Service Edition, page 127.

Mosby, *Emergency First Responder, Making the Difference*, 1st Edition, page 108.

Answer: B

9. Reference: NFPA 1001, 4.3

Brady, *First Responder*, 7th Edition, 1st Printing, page 100.

Delmar, *First Responder Handbook*, Fire Service Edition, page 83.

Mosby, *Emergency First Responder, Making the Difference*, 1st Edition, page 61.

Jones and Bartlett, AAOS, *First Responder, Your First Response in Emergency Care*, 3rd Edition, page 52.

Answer: C

10. Reference: NFPA 1001, 4.3
Brady, *First Responder*, 7th Edition, 1st Printing, page 114.
Delmar, *First Responder Handbook*, Fire Service Edition, page 134.
Mosby, *Emergency First Responder, Making the Difference*, 1st Edition, page 115.
Jones and Bartlett, AAOS, *First Responder, Your First Response in Emergency Care*, 3rd Edition, page 126.
Answer: D

11. Reference: NFPA 1001, 4.3
Brady, *First Responder*, 7th Edition, 1st Printing, page 107.
Delmar, *First Responder Handbook*, Fire Service Edition, pages 142 and 143.
Mosby, *Emergency First Responder, Making the Difference*, 1st Edition, pages 119 and 184.
Jones and Bartlett, AAOS, *First Responder, Your First Response in Emergency Care*, 3rd Edition, page 118.
Answer: D

12. Reference: NFPA 1001, 4.3
Brady, *First Responder*, 7th Edition, 1st Printing, page 99.
Delmar, *First Responder Handbook*, Fire Service Edition, page 83.
Mosby, *Emergency First Responder, Making the Difference*, 1st Edition, pages 62 and 63.
Jones and Bartlett, AAOS, *First Responder, Your First Response in Emergency Care*, 3rd Edition, page 105.
Answer: E

13. Reference: NFPA 1001, 4.3
Brady, *First Responder*, 7th Edition, 1st Printing, pages 99–100.
Delmar, *First Responder Handbook*, Fire Service Edition, page 83.
Mosby, *Emergency First Responder, Making the Difference*, 1st Edition, pages 61 and 62.
Jones and Bartlett, AAOS, *First Responder, Your First Response in Emergency Care*, 3rd Edition, pages 52–54.
Answer: D

14. Reference: NFPA 1001, 4.3
Brady, *First Responder*, 7th Edition, 1st Printing, page 113.
Delmar, *First Responder Handbook*, Fire Service Edition, page 295.
Mosby, *Emergency First Responder, Making the Difference*, 1st Edition, page 324.
Jones and Bartlett, AAOS, *First Responder, Your First Response in Emergency Care*, 3rd Edition, page 360.
Answer: D

15. Reference: NFPA 1001, 4.3
Brady, *First Responder*, 7th Edition, 1st Printing, page 285.
Delmar, *First Responder Handbook*, Fire Service Edition, page 195.
Jones and Bartlett, AAOS, *First Responder, Your First Response in Emergency Care*, 3rd Edition, page 259.
Answer: A

16. Reference: NFPA 1001, 4.3
Brady, *First Responder*, 7th Edition, 1st Printing, page 292.
Mosby, *Emergency First Responder, Making the Difference*, 1st Edition, page 241.
Answer: B

17. Reference: NFPA 1001, 4.3
Brady, *First Responder*, 7th Edition, 1st Printing, page 293.
Delmar, *First Responder Handbook*, Fire Service Edition, page 238.
Mosby, *Emergency First Responder, Making the Difference*, 1st Edition, pages 241 and 242.
Jones and Bartlett, AAOS, *First Responder, Your First Response in Emergency Care*, 3rd Edition, page 265.
Answer: C

18. Reference: NFPA 1001, 4.3
Brady, *First Responder*, 7th Edition, 1st Printing, page 302.
Mosby, *Emergency First Responder, Making the Difference*, 1st Edition, page 141.
Jones and Bartlett, AAOS, *First Responder, Your First Response in Emergency Care*, 3rd Edition, page 275.
Answer: D

19. Reference: NFPA 1001, 4.3
Brady, *First Responder*, 7th Edition, 1st Printing, page 287.
Delmar, *First Responder Handbook*, Fire Service Edition, page 235.
Mosby, *Emergency First Responder, Making the Difference*, 1st Edition, page 239.
Jones and Bartlett, AAOS, *First Responder, Your First Response in Emergency Care*, 3rd Edition, page 264.
Answer: D

20. Reference: NFPA 1001, 4.3
Brady, *First Responder*, 7th Edition, 1st Printing, pages 284–285.
Delmar, *First Responder Handbook*, Fire Service Edition, page 187.
Mosby, *Emergency First Responder, Making the Difference*, 1st Edition, pages 63 and 64.
Jones and Bartlett, AAOS, *First Responder, Your First Response in Emergency Care*, 3rd Edition, page 55.
Answer: A

21. Reference: NFPA 1001, 4.3
Brady, *First Responder*, 7th Edition, 1st Printing, page 299.
Delmar, *First Responder Handbook*, Fire Service Edition, page 237.
Mosby, *Emergency First Responder, Making the Difference*, 1st Edition, page 241.
Jones and Bartlett, AAOS, *First Responder, Your First Response in Emergency Care*, 3rd Edition, page 269.
Answer: D

22. Reference: NFPA 1001, 4.3

Brady, *First Responder*, 7th Edition, 1st Printing, page 341.

Delmar, *First Responder Handbook*, Fire Service Edition, page 243.

Mosby, *Emergency First Responder, Making the Difference*, 1st Edition, page 253.

Jones and Bartlett, AAOS, *First Responder, Your First Response in Emergency Care*, 3rd Edition, page 277.

Answer: B

23. Reference: NFPA 1001, 4.3

Brady, *First Responder*, 7th Edition, 1st Printing, page 336.

Delmar, *First Responder Handbook*, Fire Service Edition, page 241.

Mosby, *Emergency First Responder, Making the Difference*, 1st Edition, pages 249 and 252.

Jones and Bartlett, AAOS, *First Responder, Your First Response in Emergency Care*, 3rd Edition, page 274.

Answer: B

24. Reference: NFPA 1001, 4.3

Brady, *First Responder*, 7th Edition, 1st Printing, page 315.

Delmar, *First Responder Handbook*, Fire Service Edition, page 240.

Mosby, *Emergency First Responder, Making the Difference*, 1st Edition, page 247.

Jones and Bartlett, AAOS, *First Responder, Your First Response in Emergency Care*, 3rd Edition, page 267.

Answer: A

25. Reference: NFPA 1001, 4.3

Brady, *First Responder*, 7th Edition, 1st Printing, page 424.

Jones and Bartlett, AAOS, *First Responder, Your First Response in Emergency Care*, 3rd Edition, page 333.

Answer: B

26. Reference: NFPA 1001, 4.3

Brady, *First Responder*, 7th Edition, 1st Printing, page 423.

Mosby, *Emergency First Responder, Making the Difference*, 1st Edition, page 301.

Jones and Bartlett, AAOS, *First Responder, Your First Response in Emergency Care*, 3rd Edition, page 341.

Answer: B

27. Reference: NFPA 1001, 4.3

Brady, *First Responder*, 7th Edition, 1st Printing, pages 446 and 447.

Jones and Bartlett, AAOS, *First Responder, Your First Response in Emergency Care*, 3rd Edition, page 341.

Answer: D

28. Reference: NFPA 1001, 4.3

Brady, *First Responder*, 7th Edition, 1st Printing, page 422.

Delmar, *First Responder Handbook*, Fire Service Edition, page 309.

Mosby, *Emergency First Responder, Making the Difference*, 1st Edition, page 294.

Jones and Bartlett, AAOS, *First Responder, Your First Response in Emergency Care*, 3rd Edition, page 330.

Answer: C

29. Reference: NFPA 1001, 4.3

Brady, *First Responder*, 7th Edition, 1st Printing, page 423.

Delmar, *First Responder Handbook*, Fire Service Edition, pages 312 and 313.

Mosby, *Emergency First Responder, Making the Difference*, 1st Edition, page 294.

Jones and Bartlett, AAOS, *First Responder, Your First Response in Emergency Care*, 3rd Edition, page 330.

Answer: D

30. Reference: NFPA 1001, 4.3

Brady, *First Responder*, 7th Edition, 1st Printing, page 423.

Delmar, *First Responder Handbook*, Fire Service Edition, page 312.

Mosby, *Emergency First Responder, Making the Difference*, 1st Edition, page 297.

Jones and Bartlett, AAOS, *First Responder, Your First Response in Emergency Care*, 3rd Edition, page 331.

Answer: A

31. Reference: NFPA 1001, 4.3

Delmar, *First Responder Handbook*, Fire Service Edition, page 207.

Mosby, *Emergency First Responder, Making the Difference*, 1st Edition, page 199.

Jones and Bartlett, AAOS, *First Responder, Your First Response in Emergency Care*, 3rd Edition, page 447.

Answer: A

32. Reference: NFPA 1001, 4.3

Brady, *First Responder*, 7th Edition, 1st Printing, pages 206–207.

Delmar, *First Responder Handbook*, Fire Service Edition, page 210.

Mosby, *Emergency First Responder, Making the Difference*, 1st Edition, page 182.

Jones and Bartlett, AAOS, *First Responder, Your First Response in Emergency Care*, 3rd Edition, page 446.

Answer: B

33. Reference: NFPA 1001, 4.3

Brady, *First Responder*, 7th Edition, 1st Printing, page 206.

Delmar, *First Responder Handbook*, Fire Service Edition, page 212.

Mosby, *Emergency First Responder, Making the Difference*, 1st Edition, pages 199 and 200.

Jones and Bartlett, AAOS, *First Responder, Your First Response in Emergency Care*, 3rd Edition, page 448.

Answer: C

34. Reference: NFPA 1001, 4.3

Brady, *First Responder*, 7th Edition, 1st Printing, page 206.

Delmar, *First Responder Handbook*, Fire Service Edition, page 213.

Mosby, *Emergency First Responder, Making the Difference*, 1st Edition, page 198.

Answer: B

35. Reference: NFPA 1001, 4.3
Brady, *First Responder*, 7th Edition, 1st Printing, page 207.
Delmar, *First Responder Handbook*, Fire Service Edition, page 207.
Mosby, *Emergency First Responder, Making the Difference*, 1st Edition, page 198.
Jones and Bartlett, AAOS, *First Responder, Your First Response in Emergency Care*, 3rd Edition, page 449.
Answer: B

36. Reference: NFPA 1001, 4.3
Brady, *First Responder*, 7th Edition, 1st Printing, page 195.
Mosby, *Emergency First Responder, Making the Difference*, 1st Edition, page 186.
Jones and Bartlett, AAOS, *First Responder, Your First Response in Emergency Care*, 3rd Edition, page 183.
Answer: B

37. Reference: NFPA 1001, 4.3
Brady, *First Responder*, 7th Edition, 1st Printing, pages 194 and 195.
Mosby, *Emergency First Responder, Making the Difference*, 1st Edition, page 186.
Jones and Bartlett, AAOS, *First Responder, Your First Response in Emergency Care*, 3rd Edition, page 183.
Answer: D

38. Reference: NFPA 1001, 4.3
Brady, *First Responder*, 7th Edition, 1st Printing, pages 194 and 195.
Mosby, *Emergency First Responder, Making the Difference*, 1st Edition, page 186.
Jones and Bartlett, AAOS, *First Responder, Your First Response in Emergency Care*, 3rd Edition, page 183.
Answer: C

39. Reference: NFPA 1001, 4.3
Brady, *First Responder*, 7th Edition, 1st Printing, page 212.
Mosby, *Emergency First Responder, Making the Difference*, 1st Edition, page 192.
Jones and Bartlett, AAOS, *First Responder, Your First Response in Emergency Care*, 3rd Edition, page 191.
Answer: C

40. Reference: NFPA 1001, 4.3
Brady, *First Responder*, 7th Edition, 1st Printing, page 212.
Delmar, *First Responder Handbook*, Fire Service Edition, page 167.
Mosby, *Emergency First Responder, Making the Difference*, 1st Edition, page 192.
Jones and Bartlett, AAOS, *First Responder, Your First Response in Emergency Care*, 3rd Edition, page 189.
Answer: A

41. Reference: NFPA 1001, 4.3
Brady, *First Responder*, 7th Edition, 1st Printing, page 212.
Mosby, *Emergency First Responder, Making the Difference*, 1st Edition, page 184.
Jones and Bartlett, AAOS, *First Responder, Your First Response in Emergency Care*, 3rd Edition, page 190.
Answer: D

42. Reference: NFPA 1001, 4.3

Brady, *First Responder*, 7th Edition, 1st Printing, page 221.

Delmar, *First Responder Handbook*, Fire Service Edition, page 131.

Mosby, *Emergency First Responder, Making the Difference*, 1st Edition, pages 109 and 329.

Jones and Bartlett, AAOS, *First Responder, Your First Response in Emergency Care*, 3rd Edition, page 428.

Answer: B

43. Reference: NFPA 1001, 4.3

Brady, *First Responder*, 7th Edition, 1st Printing, page 204.

Delmar, *First Responder Handbook*, Fire Service Edition, page 204.

Mosby, *Emergency First Responder, Making the Difference*, 1st Edition, pages 182–183.

Jones and Bartlett, AAOS, *First Responder, Your First Response in Emergency Care*, 3rd Edition, page 446.

Answer: C

44. Reference: NFPA 1001, 4.3

Brady, *First Responder*, 7th Edition, 1st Printing, page 198.

Mosby, *Emergency First Responder, Making the Difference*, 1st Edition, page 191.

Jones and Bartlett, AAOS, *First Responder, Your First Response in Emergency Care*, 3rd Edition, page 184.

Answer: A

45. Reference: NFPA 1001, 4.3

Brady, *First Responder*, 7th Edition, 1st Printing, page 197.

Mosby, *Emergency First Responder, Making the Difference*, 1st Edition, pages 186–187.

Jones and Bartlett, AAOS, *First Responder, Your First Response in Emergency Care*, 3rd Edition, page 184.

Answer: B

46. Reference: NFPA 1001, 4.3

Brady, *First Responder*, 7th Edition, 1st Printing, page 198.

Mosby, *Emergency First Responder, Making the Difference*, 1st Edition, page 186.

Jones and Bartlett, AAOS, *First Responder, Your First Response in Emergency Care*, 3rd Edition, pages 186 and 187.

Answer: D

47. Reference: NFPA 1001, 4.3

Brady, *First Responder*, 7th Edition, 1st Printing, page 200.

Jones and Bartlett, AAOS, *First Responder, Your First Response in Emergency Care*, 3rd Edition, page 188.

Answer: B

48. Reference: NFPA 1001, 4.3

Brady, *First Responder*, 7th Edition, 1st Printing, page 55.

Delmar, *First Responder Handbook*, Fire Service Edition, page 72.

Mosby, *Emergency First Responder, Making the Difference*, 1st Edition, pages 58–59.

Jones and Bartlett, AAOS, *First Responder, Your First Response in Emergency Care*, 3rd Edition, page 51.

Answer: D

49. Reference: NFPA 1001, 4.3

Brady, *First Responder*, 7th Edition, 1st Printing, page 62.

Delmar, *First Responder Handbook*, Fire Service Edition, page 76.

Mosby, *Emergency First Responder, Making the Difference*, 1st Edition, page 69.

Jones and Bartlett, AAOS, *First Responder, Your First Response in Emergency Care*, 3rd Edition, page 59.

Answer: C

50. Reference: NFPA 1001, 4.3

Brady, *First Responder*, 7th Edition, 1st Printing, page 59.

Delmar, *First Responder Handbook*, Fire Service Edition, page 76.

Mosby, *Emergency First Responder, Making the Difference*, 1st Edition, pages 106–108.

Jones and Bartlett, AAOS, *First Responder, Your First Response in Emergency Care*, 3rd Edition, page 52.

Answer: E

51. Reference: NFPA 1001, 4.3

Brady, *First Responder*, 7th Edition, 1st Printing, page 66.

Delmar, *First Responder Handbook*, Fire Service Edition, page 186.

Mosby, *Emergency First Responder, Making the Difference*, 1st Edition, page 63.

Jones and Bartlett, AAOS, *First Responder, Your First Response in Emergency Care*, 3rd Edition, page 54.

Answer: C

52. Reference: NFPA 1001, 4.3

Brady, *First Responder*, 7th Edition, 1st Printing, page 62.

Delmar, *First Responder Handbook*, Fire Service Edition, page 76.

Mosby, *Emergency First Responder, Making the Difference*, 1st Edition, pages 69 and 70.

Jones and Bartlett, AAOS, *First Responder, Your First Response in Emergency Care*, 3rd Edition, pages 58 and 59.

Answer: B

53. Reference: NFPA 1001, 4.3

Brady, *First Responder*, 7th Edition, 1st Printing, page 61.

Delmar, *First Responder Handbook*, Fire Service Edition, pages 88–90.

Mosby, *Emergency First Responder, Making the Difference*, 1st Edition, pages 75 and 294.

Jones and Bartlett, AAOS, *First Responder, Your First Response in Emergency Care*, 3rd Edition, page 61.

Answer: E

54. Reference: NFPA 1001, 4.3

Delmar, *First Responder Handbook*, Fire Service Edition, page 92.

Mosby, *Emergency First Responder, Making the Difference*, 1st Edition, page 76.

Jones and Bartlett, AAOS, *First Responder, Your First Response in Emergency Care*, 3rd Edition, page 62.

Answer: C

55. Reference: NFPA 1001, 4.3
Brady, *First Responder*, 7th Edition, 1st Printing, page 61.
Delmar, *First Responder Handbook*, Fire Service Edition, pages 123–125.
Mosby, *Emergency First Responder, Making the Difference*, 1st Edition, page 60.
Jones and Bartlett, AAOS, *First Responder, Your First Response in Emergency Care*, 3rd Edition, page 52.
Answer: D

56. Reference: NFPA 1001, 4.3
Brady, *First Responder*, 7th Edition, 1st Printing, pages 54–55.
Delmar, *First Responder Handbook*, Fire Service Edition, page 72.
Mosby, *Emergency First Responder, Making the Difference*, 1st Edition, page 57.
Jones and Bartlett, AAOS, *First Responder, Your First Response in Emergency Care*, 3rd Edition, page 72.
Answer: C

57. Reference: NFPA 1001, 4.3
Brady, *First Responder*, 7th Edition, 1st Printing, page 55.
Delmar, *First Responder Handbook*, Fire Service Edition, page 72.
Mosby, *Emergency First Responder, Making the Difference*, 1st Edition, page 58.
Jones and Bartlett, AAOS, *First Responder, Your First Response in Emergency Care*, 3rd Edition, page 50.
Answer: A

58. Reference: NFPA 1001, 4.3
Brady, *First Responder*, 7th Edition, 1st Printing, page 55.
Delmar, *First Responder Handbook*, Fire Service Edition, page 72.
Mosby, *Emergency First Responder, Making the Difference*, 1st Edition, page 59.
Jones and Bartlett, AAOS, *First Responder, Your First Response in Emergency Care*, 3rd Edition, page 51.
Answer: D

59. Reference: NFPA 1001, 4.3
Brady, *First Responder*, 7th Edition, 1st Printing, page 58.
Delmar, *First Responder Handbook*, Fire Service Edition, page 79.
Mosby, *Emergency First Responder, Making the Difference*, 1st Edition, page 60.
Jones and Bartlett, AAOS, *First Responder, Your First Response in Emergency Care*, 3rd Edition, page 57.
Answer: B

60. Reference: NFPA 1001, 4.3
Brady, *First Responder*, 7th Edition, 1st Printing, page 461.
Mosby, *Emergency First Responder, Making the Difference*, 1st Edition, pages 316–317 and 319.
Answer: B

61. Reference: NFPA 1001, 4.3
Brady, *First Responder*, 7th Edition, 1st Printing, page 464.
Answer: B

62. Reference: NFPA 1001, 4.3
Brady, *First Responder*, 7th Edition, 1st Printing, pages 477 and 478.
Delmar, *First Responder Handbook*, Fire Service Edition, page 300.
Mosby, *Emergency First Responder, Making the Difference*, 1st Edition, page 328.
Jones and Bartlett, AAOS, *First Responder, Your First Response in Emergency Care*, 3rd Edition, page 367.
Answer: A

63. Reference: NFPA 1001, 4.3
Brady, *First Responder*, 7th Edition, 1st Printing, page 491.
Delmar, *First Responder Handbook*, Fire Service Edition, page 304.
Mosby, *Emergency First Responder, Making the Difference*, 1st Edition, page 329.
Jones and Bartlett, AAOS, *First Responder, Your First Response in Emergency Care*, 3rd Edition, page 371.
Answer: C

64. Reference: NFPA 1001, 4.3
Brady, *First Responder*, 7th Edition, 1st Printing, pages 461–466.
Delmar, *First Responder Handbook*, Fire Service Edition, pages 292–294.
Mosby, *Emergency First Responder, Making the Difference*, 1st Edition, pages 187 and 317.
Jones and Bartlett, AAOS, *First Responder, Your First Response in Emergency Care*, 3rd Edition, page 349.
Answer: B

65. Reference: NFPA 1001, 4.3
Brady, *First Responder*, 7th Edition, 1st Printing, page 6.
Delmar, *First Responder Handbook*, Fire Service Edition, pages 57–58.
Mosby, *Emergency First Responder, Making the Difference*, 1st Edition, page 42.
Jones and Bartlett, AAOS, *First Responder, Your First Response in Emergency Care*, 3rd Edition, page 37.
Answer: B

66. Reference: NFPA 1001, 4.3
Brady, *First Responder*, 7th Edition, 1st Printing, page 5.
Delmar, *First Responder Handbook*, Fire Service Edition, page 18.
Mosby, *Emergency First Responder, Making the Difference*, 1st Edition, page 11.
Jones and Bartlett, AAOS, *First Responder, Your First Response in Emergency Care*, 3rd Edition, page 15.
Answer: D

67. Reference: NFPA 1001, 4.3
Brady, *First Responder*, 7th Edition, 1st Printing, page 5.
Delmar, *First Responder Handbook*, Fire Service Edition, pages 18–19.
Mosby, *Emergency First Responder, Making the Difference*, 1st Edition, page 12.
Jones and Bartlett, AAOS, *First Responder, Your First Response in Emergency Care*, 3rd Edition, page 15.
Answer: A

68. Reference: NFPA 1001, 4.3

Brady, *First Responder*, 7th Edition, 1st Printing, page 5.

Delmar, *First Responder Handbook*, Fire Service Edition, pages 18–19.

Mosby, *Emergency First Responder, Making the Difference*, 1st Edition, page 12.

Jones and Bartlett, AAOS, *First Responder, Your First Response in Emergency Care*, 3rd Edition, page 15.

Answer: A

69. Reference: NFPA 1001, 4.3

Brady, *First Responder*, 7th Edition, 1st Printing, page 3.

Delmar, *First Responder Handbook*, Fire Service Edition, page 3.

Mosby, *Emergency First Responder, Making the Difference*, 1st Edition, page 7.

Jones and Bartlett, AAOS, *First Responder, Your First Response in Emergency Care*, 3rd Edition, page 4.

Answer: B

70. Reference: NFPA 1001, 4.3

Brady, *First Responder*, 7th Edition, 1st Printing, page 3.

Answer: C

71. Reference: NFPA 1001, 4.3

Brady, *First Responder*, 7th Edition, 1st Printing, pages 8 and 44.

Delmar, *First Responder Handbook*, Fire Service Edition, pages 42–49.

Mosby, *Emergency First Responder, Making the Difference*, 1st Edition, pages 27 and 30.

Jones and Bartlett, AAOS, *First Responder, Your First Response in Emergency Care*, 3rd Edition, page 335.

Answer: D

72. Reference: NFPA 1001, 4.3

Brady, *First Responder*, 7th Edition, 1st Printing, page 8.

Delmar, *First Responder Handbook*, Fire Service Edition, page 37.

Mosby, *Emergency First Responder, Making the Difference*, 1st Edition, pages 9 and 32.

Jones and Bartlett, AAOS, *First Responder, Your First Response in Emergency Care*, 3rd Edition, page 27.

Answer: D

73. Reference: NFPA 1001, 4.3

Brady, *First Responder*, 7th Edition, 1st Printing, page 22.

Delmar, *First Responder Handbook*, Fire Service Edition, page 59.

Mosby, *Emergency First Responder, Making the Difference*, 1st Edition, page 43.

Jones and Bartlett, AAOS, *First Responder, Your First Response in Emergency Care*, 3rd Edition, page 37.

Answer: B

74. Reference: NFPA 1001, 4.3

Brady, *First Responder*, 7th Edition, 1st Printing, page 21.

Delmar, *First Responder Handbook*, Fire Service Edition, page 59.

Mosby, *Emergency First Responder, Making the Difference*, 1st Edition, page 44.

Jones and Bartlett, AAOS, *First Responder, Your First Response in Emergency Care*, 3rd Edition, page 39.

Answer: D

75. Reference: NFPA 1001, 4.3
Brady, *First Responder*, 7th Edition, 1st Printing, page 25.
Delmar, *First Responder Handbook*, Fire Service Edition, page 61.
Mosby, *Emergency First Responder, Making the Difference*, 1st Edition, page 48.
Jones and Bartlett, AAOS, *First Responder, Your First Response in Emergency Care*, 3rd Edition, page 41.
Answer: E

76. Reference: NFPA 1001, 4.3
Brady, *First Responder*, 7th Edition, 1st Printing, pages 19 and 20.
Mosby, *Emergency First Responder, Making the Difference*, 1st Edition, page 42.
Jones and Bartlett, AAOS, *First Responder, Your First Response in Emergency Care*, 3rd Edition, page 36.
Answer: D

77. Reference: NFPA 1001, 4.3
Brady, *First Responder*, 7th Edition, 1st Printing, page 23.
Delmar, *First Responder Handbook*, Fire Service Edition, page 60.
Mosby, *Emergency First Responder, Making the Difference*, 1st Edition, page 45.
Jones and Bartlett, AAOS, *First Responder, Your First Response in Emergency Care*, 3rd Edition, page 38.
Answer: B

78. Reference: NFPA 1001, 4.3
Brady, *First Responder*, 7th Edition, 1st Printing, page 29.
Delmar, *First Responder Handbook*, Fire Service Edition, pages 167 and 168.
Mosby, *Emergency First Responder, Making the Difference*, 1st Edition, page 50.
Jones and Bartlett, AAOS, *First Responder, Your First Response in Emergency Care*, 3rd Edition, page 215, Fig. 9.8.
Answer: B

79. Reference: NFPA 1001, 4.3
Brady, *First Responder*, 7th Edition, 1st Printing, page 70.
Delmar, *First Responder Handbook*, Fire Service Edition, page 100.
Mosby, *Emergency First Responder, Making the Difference*, 1st Edition, page 84.
Jones and Bartlett, AAOS, *First Responder, Your First Response in Emergency Care*, 3rd Edition, page 69.
Answer: A

80. Reference: NFPA 1001, 4.3
Brady, *First Responder*, 7th Edition, 1st Printing, pages 83–85.
Delmar, *First Responder Handbook*, Fire Service Edition, page 118.
Mosby, *Emergency First Responder, Making the Difference*, 1st Edition, pages 97 and 98.
Jones and Bartlett, AAOS, *First Responder, Your First Response in Emergency Care*, 3rd Edition, pages 81–83.
Answer: E

81. Reference: NFPA 1001, 4.3
Brady, *First Responder*, 7th Edition, 1st Printing, page 80.
Delmar, *First Responder Handbook*, Fire Service Edition, page 103.
Mosby, *Emergency First Responder, Making the Difference*, 1st Edition, page 93.
Answer: A

82. Reference: NFPA 1001, 4.3
Brady, *First Responder*, 7th Edition, 1st Printing, pages 70–72.
Delmar, *First Responder Handbook*, Fire Service Edition, page 103.
Mosby, *Emergency First Responder, Making the Difference*, 1st Edition, page 85.
Jones and Bartlett, AAOS, *First Responder, Your First Response in Emergency Care*, 3rd Edition, page 70.
Answer: B

83. Reference: NFPA 1001, 4.3
Brady, *First Responder*, 7th Edition, 1st Printing, page 69.
Delmar, *First Responder Handbook*, Fire Service Edition, page 100.
Mosby, *Emergency First Responder, Making the Difference*, 1st Edition, page 84.
Jones and Bartlett, AAOS, *First Responder, Your First Response in Emergency Care*, 3rd Edition, page 69.
Answer: C

84. Reference: NFPA 1001, 4.3
Brady, *First Responder*, 7th Edition, 1st Printing, page 71.
Delmar, *First Responder Handbook*, Fire Service Edition, page 103.
Mosby, *Emergency First Responder, Making the Difference*, 1st Edition, page 87.
Jones and Bartlett, AAOS, *First Responder, Your First Response in Emergency Care*, 3rd Edition, page 70.
Answer: A

85. Reference: NFPA 1001, 4.3
Brady, *First Responder*, 7th Edition, 1st Printing, page 71.
Delmar, *First Responder Handbook*, Fire Service Edition, page 103.
Mosby, *Emergency First Responder, Making the Difference*, 1st Edition, page 87.
Jones and Bartlett, AAOS, *First Responder, Your First Response in Emergency Care*, 3rd Edition, page 70.
Answer: B

86. Reference: NFPA 1001, 4.3
Brady, *First Responder*, 7th Edition, 1st Printing, page 71.
Delmar, *First Responder Handbook*, Fire Service Edition, pages 103 and 104.
Mosby, *Emergency First Responder, Making the Difference*, 1st Edition, page 88.
Jones and Bartlett, AAOS, *First Responder, Your First Response in Emergency Care*, 3rd Edition, pages 70–72.
Answer: C

87. Reference: NFPA 1001, 4.3
Brady, *First Responder*, 7th Edition, 1st Printing, page 78.
Mosby, *Emergency First Responder, Making the Difference*, 1st Edition, page 93.
Jones and Bartlett, AAOS, *First Responder, Your First Response in Emergency Care*, 3rd Edition, page 69.
Answer: A

88. Reference: NFPA 1001, 4.3

Brady, *First Responder*, 7th Edition, 1st Printing, page 82.

Delmar, *First Responder Handbook*, Fire Service Edition, page 272.

Mosby, *Emergency First Responder, Making the Difference*, 1st Edition, page 283.

Jones and Bartlett, AAOS, *First Responder, Your First Response in Emergency Care*, 3rd Edition, page 84.

Answer: B

89. Reference: NFPA 1001, 4.3

Brady, *First Responder*, 7th Edition, 1st Printing, page 266.

Delmar, *First Responder Handbook*, Fire Service Edition, pages 222–223.

Mosby, *Emergency First Responder, Making the Difference*, 1st Edition, page 221.

Jones and Bartlett, AAOS, *First Responder, Your First Response in Emergency Care*, 3rd Edition, page 209.

Answer: B

90. Reference: NFPA 1001, 4.3

Brady, *First Responder*, 7th Edition, 1st Printing, page 269.

Delmar, *First Responder Handbook*, Fire Service Edition, pages 223–224.

Mosby, *Emergency First Responder, Making the Difference*, 1st Edition, page 220.

Jones and Bartlett, AAOS, *First Responder, Your First Response in Emergency Care*, 3rd Edition, page 208.

Answer: A

91. Reference: NFPA 1001, 4.3

Brady, *First Responder*, 7th Edition, 1st Printing, page 269.

Delmar, *First Responder Handbook*, Fire Service Edition, page 224.

Mosby, *Emergency First Responder, Making the Difference*, 1st Edition, page 220.

Jones and Bartlett, AAOS, *First Responder, Your First Response in Emergency Care*, 3rd Edition, page 209.

Answer: A

92. Reference: NFPA 1001, 4.3

Brady, *First Responder*, 7th Edition, 1st Printing, pages 265 and 266.

Delmar, *First Responder Handbook*, Fire Service Edition, pages 224–225.

Mosby, *Emergency First Responder, Making the Difference*, 1st Edition, pages 223 and 224.

Jones and Bartlett, AAOS, *First Responder, Your First Response in Emergency Care*, 3rd Edition, page 207.

Answer: C

93. Reference: NFPA 1001, 4.3

Brady, *First Responder*, 7th Edition, 1st Printing, pages 245–246.

Mosby, *Emergency First Responder, Making the Difference*, 1st Edition, page 218.

Jones and Bartlett, AAOS, *First Responder, Your First Response in Emergency Care*, 3rd Edition, page 214.

Answer: A

94. Reference: NFPA 1001, 4.3
Brady, *First Responder*, 7th Edition, 1st Printing, pages 244 and 245.
Mosby, *Emergency First Responder, Making the Difference*, 1st Edition, page 219.
Jones and Bartlett, AAOS, *First Responder, Your First Response in Emergency Care*, 3rd Edition, page 214.
Answer: C

95. Reference: NFPA 1001, 4.3
Brady, *First Responder*, 7th Edition, 1st Printing, page 239.
Answer: A

96. Reference: NFPA 1001, 4.3
Brady, *First Responder*, 7th Edition, 1st Printing, page 528.
Delmar, *First Responder Handbook*, Fire Service Edition, pages 160, 327, and 340.
Mosby, *Emergency First Responder, Making the Difference*, 1st Edition, pages 166 and 351.
Jones and Bartlett, AAOS, *First Responder, Your First Response in Emergency Care*, 3rd Edition, page 400.
Answer: D

97. Reference: NFPA 1001, 4.3
Brady, *First Responder*, 7th Edition, 1st Printing, page 527.
Delmar, *First Responder Handbook*, Fire Service Edition, page 341.
Mosby, *Emergency First Responder, Making the Difference*, 1st Edition, page 343.
Jones and Bartlett, AAOS, *First Responder, Your First Response in Emergency Care*, 3rd Edition, page 406.
Answer: D

98. Reference: NFPA 1001, 4.3
Brady, *First Responder*, 7th Edition, 1st Printing, page 418.
Delmar, *First Responder Handbook*, Fire Service Edition, page 284.
Mosby, *Emergency First Responder, Making the Difference*, 1st Edition, pages 275 and 287.
Jones and Bartlett, AAOS, *First Responder, Your First Response in Emergency Care*, 3rd Edition, pages 311 and 313.
Answer: B

99. Reference: NFPA 1001, 4.3
Brady, *First Responder*, 7th Edition, 1st Printing, page 397.
Delmar, *First Responder Handbook*, Fire Service Edition, pages 285–286.
Mosby, *Emergency First Responder, Making the Difference*, 1st Edition, page 291, Box 11-6.
Jones and Bartlett, AAOS, *First Responder, Your First Response in Emergency Care*, 3rd Edition, page 310.
Answer: D

100. Reference: NFPA 1001, 4.3
Brady, *First Responder*, 7th Edition, 1st Printing, page 396.
Jones and Bartlett, AAOS, *First Responder, Your First Response in Emergency Care*, 3rd Edition, page 267.
Answer: D

101. Reference: NFPA 1001, 4.3

Brady, *First Responder*, 7th Edition, 1st Printing, page 370.

Mosby, *Emergency First Responder, Making the Difference*, 1st Edition, pages 270–271.

Answer: A

102. Reference: NFPA 1001, 4.3

Brady, *First Responder*, 7th Edition, 1st Printing, page 361.

Mosby, *Emergency First Responder, Making the Difference*, 1st Edition, pages 268–269.

Jones and Bartlett, AAOS, *First Responder, Your First Response in Emergency Care*, 3rd Edition, page 291.

Answer: A

103. Reference: NFPA 1001, 4.3

Brady, *First Responder*, 7th Edition, 1st Printing, page 370.

Answer: C

104. Reference: NFPA 1001, 4.3

Brady, *First Responder*, 7th Edition, 1st Printing, page 360.

Delmar, *First Responder Handbook*, Fire Service Edition, page 257.

Mosby, *Emergency First Responder, Making the Difference*, 1st Edition, page 269.

Jones and Bartlett, AAOS, *First Responder, Your First Response in Emergency Care*, 3rd Edition, page 292.

Answer: B

105. Reference: NFPA 1001, 4.3

Brady, *First Responder*, 7th Edition, 1st Printing, page 401.

Delmar, *First Responder Handbook*, Fire Service Edition, pages 283–284.

Mosby, *Emergency First Responder, Making the Difference*, 1st Edition, page 279.

Jones and Bartlett, AAOS, *First Responder, Your First Response in Emergency Care*, 3rd Edition, page 315.

Answer: D

106. Reference: NFPA 1001, 4.3

Brady, *First Responder*, 7th Edition, 1st Printing, page 393.

Delmar, *First Responder Handbook*, Fire Service Edition, page 76.

Mosby, *Emergency First Responder, Making the Difference*, 1st Edition, page 69.

Jones and Bartlett, AAOS, *First Responder, Your First Response in Emergency Care*, 3rd Edition, page 58.

Answer: E

107. Reference: NFPA 1001, 4.3

Brady, *First Responder*, 7th Edition, 1st Printing, page 141.

Mosby, *Emergency First Responder, Making the Difference*, 1st Edition, page 140.

Jones and Bartlett, AAOS, *First Responder, Your First Response in Emergency Care*, 3rd Edition, page 147.

Answer: C

108. Reference: NFPA 1001, 4.3
Brady, *First Responder*, 7th Edition, 1st Printing, page 164.
Delmar, *First Responder Handbook*, Fire Service Edition, pages 179 and 180.
Mosby, *Emergency First Responder, Making the Difference*, 1st Edition, page 162.
Jones and Bartlett, AAOS, *First Responder, Your First Response in Emergency Care*, 3rd Edition, page 216.
Answer: B

109. Reference: NFPA 1001, 4.3
Brady, *First Responder*, 7th Edition, 1st Printing, page 178.
Delmar, *First Responder Handbook*, Fire Service Edition, page 180.
Mosby, *Emergency First Responder, Making the Difference*, 1st Edition, page 162.
Jones and Bartlett, AAOS, *First Responder, Your First Response in Emergency Care*, 3rd Edition, page 163.
Answer: C

110. Reference: NFPA 1001, 4.3
Brady, *First Responder*, 7th Edition, 1st Printing, page 168.
Delmar, *First Responder Handbook*, Fire Service Edition, page 175.
Mosby, *Emergency First Responder, Making the Difference*, 1st Edition, pages 22 and 163.
Answer: E

111. Reference: NFPA 1001, 4.3
Brady, *First Responder*, 7th Edition, 1st Printing, page 159.
Mosby, *Emergency First Responder, Making the Difference*, 1st Edition, page 142, Table 7-9.
Jones and Bartlett, AAOS, *First Responder, Your First Response in Emergency Care*, 3rd Edition, page 152.
Answer: B

112. Reference: NFPA 1001, 4.3
Delmar, *First Responder Handbook*, Fire Service Edition, page 169.
Mosby, *Emergency First Responder, Making the Difference*, 1st Edition, page 154.
Jones and Bartlett, AAOS, *First Responder, Your First Response in Emergency Care*, 3rd Edition, page 155.
Answer: D

113. Reference: NFPA 1001, 4.3
Brady, *First Responder*, 7th Edition, 1st Printing, pages 143 and 157.
Delmar, *First Responder Handbook*, Fire Service Edition, page 168.
Mosby, *Emergency First Responder, Making the Difference*, 1st Edition, page 151.
Jones and Bartlett, AAOS, *First Responder, Your First Response in Emergency Care*, 3rd Edition, page 294.
Answer: C

114. Reference: NFPA 1001, 4.3
Brady, *First Responder*, 7th Edition, 1st Printing, page 157.
Delmar, *First Responder Handbook*, Fire Service Edition, page 295.
Mosby, *Emergency First Responder, Making the Difference*, 1st Edition, page 322.
Jones and Bartlett, AAOS, *First Responder, Your First Response in Emergency Care*, 3rd Edition, page 351.
Answer: E

115. Reference: NFPA 1001, 4.3
Brady, *First Responder*, 7th Edition, 1st Printing, pages 335 and 337.
Delmar, *First Responder Handbook*, Fire Service Edition, page 165.
Mosby, *Emergency First Responder, Making the Difference*, 1st Edition, page 159.
Jones and Bartlett, AAOS, *First Responder, Your First Response in Emergency Care*, 3rd Edition, pages 274 and 321.
Answer: A

116. Reference: NFPA 1001, 4.3
Brady, *First Responder*, 7th Edition, 1st Printing, page 585.
Delmar, *First Responder Handbook*, Fire Service Edition, page 218.
Mosby, *Emergency First Responder, Making the Difference*, 1st Edition, page 365.
Answer: B

117. Reference: NFPA 1001, 4.3
Delmar, *First Responder Handbook*, Fire Service Edition, page 226.
Mosby, *Emergency First Responder, Making the Difference*, 1st Edition, page 226.
Jones and Bartlett, AAOS, *First Responder, Your First Response in Emergency Care*, 3rd Edition, page 238.
Answer: E

118. Reference: NFPA 1001, 4.3
Brady, *First Responder*, 7th Edition, 1st Printing, pages 264 and 265.
Delmar, *First Responder Handbook*, Fire Service Edition, page 225.
Mosby, *Emergency First Responder, Making the Difference*, 1st Edition, page 223, Table 9-4, and page 224.
Jones and Bartlett, AAOS, *First Responder, Your First Response in Emergency Care*, 3rd Edition, page 207.
Answer: B

119. Reference: NFPA 1001, 4.3
Brady, *First Responder*, 7th Edition, 1st Printing, page 246.
Delmar, *First Responder Handbook*, Fire Service Edition, page 221.
Mosby, *Emergency First Responder, Making the Difference*, 1st Edition, page 217.
Jones and Bartlett, AAOS, *First Responder, Your First Response in Emergency Care*, 3rd Edition, page 204.
Answer: A

120. Reference: NFPA 1001, 4.3

Brady, *First Responder*, 7th Edition, 1st Printing, page 157.

Delmar, *First Responder Handbook*, Fire Service Edition, page 296.

Mosby, *Emergency First Responder, Making the Difference*, 1st Edition, page 324.

Jones and Bartlett, AAOS, *First Responder, Your First Response in Emergency Care*, 3rd Edition, pages 152 and 351.

Answer: A

121. Reference: NFPA 1001, 4.3

Brady, *First Responder*, 7th Edition, 1st Printing, page 48.

Delmar, *First Responder Handbook*, Fire Service Edition, pages 157 and 335.

Mosby, *Emergency First Responder, Making the Difference*, 1st Edition, pages 139–144.

Jones and Bartlett, AAOS, *First Responder, Your First Response in Emergency Care*, 3rd Edition, pages 386–387.

Answer: C

122. Reference: NFPA 1001, 4.3

Brady, *First Responder*, 7th Edition, 1st Printing, page 38.

Mosby, *Emergency First Responder, Making the Difference*, 1st Edition, page 48.

Jones and Bartlett, AAOS, *First Responder, Your First Response in Emergency Care*, 3rd Edition, page 42.

Answer: A

123. Reference: NFPA 1001, 4.3

Brady, *First Responder*, 7th Edition, 1st Printing, page 39.

Delmar, *First Responder Handbook*, Fire Service Edition, page 26.

Mosby, *Emergency First Responder, Making the Difference*, 1st Edition, pages 24–25.

Jones and Bartlett, AAOS, *First Responder, Your First Response in Emergency Care*, 3rd Edition, page 24.

Answer: C

124. Reference: NFPA 1001, 4.3

Brady, *First Responder*, 7th Edition, 1st Printing, page 39.

Delmar, *First Responder Handbook*, Fire Service Edition, page 26.

Mosby, *Emergency First Responder, Making the Difference*, 1st Edition, page 24.

Jones and Bartlett, AAOS, *First Responder, Your First Response in Emergency Care*, 3rd Edition, page 22.

Answer: E

125. Reference: NFPA 1001, 4.3

Brady, *First Responder*, 7th Edition, 1st Printing, page 39.

Delmar, *First Responder Handbook*, Fire Service Edition, page 30.

Mosby, *Emergency First Responder, Making the Difference*, 1st Edition, page 23.

Jones and Bartlett, AAOS, *First Responder, Your First Response in Emergency Care*, 3rd Edition, page 21.

Answer: C

126. Reference: NFPA 1001, 4.3
Brady, *First Responder*, 7th Edition, 1st Printing, page 39.
Delmar, *First Responder Handbook*, Fire Service Edition, page 30.
Mosby, *Emergency First Responder, Making the Difference*, 1st Edition, page 23.
Jones and Bartlett, AAOS, *First Responder, Your First Response in Emergency Care*, 3rd Edition, page 21.
Answer: B

127. Reference: NFPA 1001, 4.3
Brady, *First Responder*, 7th Edition, 1st Printing, page 41.
Delmar, *First Responder Handbook*, Fire Service Edition, page 31.
Mosby, *Emergency First Responder, Making the Difference*, 1st Edition, page 25.
Jones and Bartlett, AAOS, *First Responder, Your First Response in Emergency Care*, 3rd Edition, page 10.
Answer: D

128. Reference: NFPA 1001, 4.3
Delmar, *First Responder Handbook*, Fire Service Edition, pages 31–32.
Mosby, *Emergency First Responder, Making the Difference*, 1st Edition, page 26.
Jones and Bartlett, AAOS, *First Responder, Your First Response in Emergency Care*, 3rd Edition, page 371.
Answer: D

129. Reference: NFPA 1001, 4.3
Delmar, *First Responder Handbook*, Fire Service Edition, page 31.
Mosby, *Emergency First Responder, Making the Difference*, 1st Edition, page 25.
Jones and Bartlett, AAOS, *First Responder, Your First Response in Emergency Care*, 3rd Edition, pages 248–249.
Answer: A

130. Reference: NFPA 1001, 4.3
Brady, *First Responder*, 7th Edition, 1st Printing, page 41.
Delmar, *First Responder Handbook*, Fire Service Edition, page 32.
Mosby, *Emergency First Responder, Making the Difference*, 1st Edition, page 26, Box 2-3.
Jones and Bartlett, AAOS, *First Responder, Your First Response in Emergency Care*, 3rd Edition, page 25.
Answer: B

131. Reference: NFPA 1001, 4.3
Brady, *First Responder*, 7th Edition, 1st Printing, pages 36, 37, and 41.
Delmar, *First Responder Handbook*, Fire Service Edition, pages 31–33.
Mosby, *Emergency First Responder, Making the Difference*, 1st Edition, page 25.
Jones and Bartlett, AAOS, *First Responder, Your First Response in Emergency Care*, 3rd Edition, page 25.
Answer: E

132. Reference: NFPA 1001, 4.3
Brady, *First Responder*, 7th Edition, 1st Printing, pages 8 and 36–37.
Delmar, *First Responder Handbook*, Fire Service Edition, pages 24–49.
Mosby, *Emergency First Responder, Making the Difference*, 1st Edition, pages 24, 26, and 31.
Jones and Bartlett, AAOS, *First Responder, Your First Response in Emergency Care*, 3rd Edition, pages 25–27.
Answer: B

133. Reference: NFPA 1001, 4.3
Brady, *First Responder*, 7th Edition, 1st Printing, page 43.
Delmar, *First Responder Handbook*, Fire Service Edition, page 42.
Answer: B

134. Reference: NFPA 1001, 4.3
Brady, *First Responder*, 7th Edition, 1st Printing, page 39.
Mosby, *Emergency First Responder, Making the Difference*, 1st Edition, page 24.
Jones and Bartlett, AAOS, *First Responder, Your First Response in Emergency Care*, 3rd Edition, page 242.
Answer: A

135. Reference: NFPA 1001, 4.3
Brady, *First Responder*, 7th Edition, 1st Printing, page 42.
Delmar, *First Responder Handbook*, Fire Service Edition, page 42.
Mosby, *Emergency First Responder, Making the Difference*, 1st Edition, page 26.
Jones and Bartlett, AAOS, *First Responder, Your First Response in Emergency Care*, 3rd Edition, page 26.
Answer: A

136. Reference: NFPA 1001, 4.3
Brady, *First Responder*, 7th Edition, 1st Printing, page 39.
Delmar, *First Responder Handbook*, Fire Service Edition, page 26.
Mosby, *Emergency First Responder, Making the Difference*, 1st Edition, page 24.
Jones and Bartlett, AAOS, *First Responder, Your First Response in Emergency Care*, 3rd Edition, page 22.
Answer: D

137. Reference: NFPA 1001, 4.3
Brady, *First Responder*, 7th Edition, 1st Printing, pages 44 and 191.
Delmar, *First Responder Handbook*, Fire Service Edition, pages 42–49.
Mosby, *Emergency First Responder, Making the Difference*, 1st Edition, pages 26 and 115.
Jones and Bartlett, AAOS, *First Responder, Your First Response in Emergency Care*, 3rd Edition, pages 26–27.
Answer: C

138. Reference: NFPA 1001, 4.3
Delmar, *First Responder Handbook*, Fire Service Edition, page 45.
Answer: D

139. Reference: NFPA 1001, 4.3
Brady, *First Responder*, 7th Edition, 1st Printing, page 47.
Delmar, *First Responder Handbook*, Fire Service Edition, pages 50–51.
Jones and Bartlett, AAOS, *First Responder, Your First Response in Emergency Care*, 3rd Edition, page 27.
Answer: D

140. Reference: NFPA 1001, 4.3
Delmar, *First Responder Handbook*, Fire Service Edition, page 44.
Jones and Bartlett, AAOS, *First Responder, Your First Response in Emergency Care*, 3rd Edition, page 26.
Answer: A

141. Reference: NFPA 1001, 4.3
Delmar, *First Responder Handbook*, Fire Service Edition, page 49.
Mosby, *Emergency First Responder, Making the Difference*, 1st Edition, page 27.
Jones and Bartlett, AAOS, *First Responder, Your First Response in Emergency Care*, 3rd Edition, page 26.
Answer: C

142. Reference: NFPA 1001, 4.3
Brady, *First Responder*, 7th Edition, 1st Printing, pages 43 and 45.
Delmar, *First Responder Handbook*, Fire Service Edition, page 41.
Answer: C

143. Reference: NFPA 1001, 4.3
Brady, *First Responder*, 7th Edition, 1st Printing, page 44.
Delmar, *First Responder Handbook*, Fire Service Edition, page 48.
Mosby, *Emergency First Responder, Making the Difference*, 1st Edition, pages 27 and 29.
Jones and Bartlett, AAOS, *First Responder, Your First Response in Emergency Care*, 3rd Edition, page 27.
Answer: A

144. Reference: NFPA 1001, 4.3
Brady, *First Responder*, 7th Edition, 1st Printing, page 44.
Delmar, *First Responder Handbook*, Fire Service Edition, page 48.
Mosby, *Emergency First Responder, Making the Difference*, 1st Edition, page 27.
Jones and Bartlett, AAOS, *First Responder, Your First Response in Emergency Care*, 3rd Edition, page 27.
Answer: D

145. Reference: NFPA 1001, 4.3
Brady, *First Responder*, 7th Edition, 1st Printing, page 44.
Delmar, *First Responder Handbook*, Fire Service Edition, page 39.
Mosby, *Emergency First Responder, Making the Difference*, 1st Edition, page 27.
Jones and Bartlett, AAOS, *First Responder, Your First Response in Emergency Care*, 3rd Edition, page 27.
Answer: C

146. Reference: NFPA 1001, 4.3
Brady, *First Responder*, 7th Edition, 1st Printing, page 45.
Delmar, *First Responder Handbook*, Fire Service Edition, page 46.
Mosby, *Emergency First Responder, Making the Difference*, 1st Edition, page 240.
Jones and Bartlett, AAOS, *First Responder, Your First Response in Emergency Care*, 3rd Edition, page 26.
Answer: E

147. Reference: NFPA 1001, 4.3
Brady, *First Responder*, 7th Edition, 1st Printing, page 45.
Delmar, *First Responder Handbook*, Fire Service Edition, page 44.
Jones and Bartlett, AAOS, *First Responder, Your First Response in Emergency Care*, 3rd Edition, page 26.
Answer: B

148. Reference: NFPA 1001, 4.3
Delmar, *First Responder Handbook*, Fire Service Edition, pages 39–40.
Mosby, *Emergency First Responder, Making the Difference*, 1st Edition, page 27.
Answer: E

149. Reference: NFPA 1001, 4.3
Delmar, *First Responder Handbook*, Fire Service Edition, page 44.
Answer: D

150. Reference: NFPA 1001, 4.3
Brady, *First Responder*, 7th Edition, 1st Printing, page 44.
Delmar, *First Responder Handbook*, Fire Service Edition, page 42.
Mosby, *Emergency First Responder, Making the Difference*, 1st Edition, page 27.
Jones and Bartlett, AAOS, *First Responder, Your First Response in Emergency Care*, 3rd Edition, page 26.
Answer: A

Don't forget to enter the information on your Personal Progress Plotter and answer the Yes and No question at the end of the Examination. This step is extremely important for the successful completion of the Systematic Approach to Examination Preparation!

BIBLIOGRAPHY FOR EXAM PREP: Medical First Responder

1. DOT, First Responder National Standard Curriculum

2. NFPA 1001, Professional Qualifications for Firefighter I and II, 2002

3. Brady, *First Responder*, 7th Edition

4. Delmar, *First Responder Handbook*, Fire Service Edition

5. Mosby, *Emergency First Responder, Making the Difference*, 1st Edition

6. Jones and Bartlett, AAOS, *First Responder, Your First Response in Emergency Care*, 3rd Edition

Performance Training Systems, Inc.
Training and testing that are on target!

Online examinations for the Fire and Emergency Medical Services

Registration

FREE OFFER - 150 ITEM PRACTICE TEST - VALUED AT $39.00

Complete registration form and fax it to (561) 863-1386.

_____
Name

_____
Title

_____
Department

_____
Address: Street

_____
City   State   Zip Code

_____
Telephone   Fax

_____
E-mail

Choose the tests that apply to your needs.

- ☐ Aerial Operator
- ☐ Airport Fire Fighter
- ☐ Confined Space Rescue
- ☐ EMT-Basic
- ☐ Fire and Life Safety Educator 1
- ☐ Fire and Life Safety Educator 2
- ☐ Fire Department Safety Officer
- ☐ Fire Fighter 1
- ☐ Fire Fighter 2

- ☐ Fire Inspector 1
- ☐ Fire Inspector 2
- ☐ Fire Instructor 1
- ☐ Fire Instructor 2
- ☐ Fire Investigator
- ☐ Fire Officer 1
- ☐ Fire Officer 2
- ☐ HazMat Awareness
- ☐ HazMat Operations
- ☐ HazMat Technician
- ☐ Medical First Responder

- ☐ Pumper Driver
- ☐ Ropes and Rigging Rescue
- ☐ Structural Collapse Rescue
- ☐ Vehicle/Machinery Rescue
- ☐ Water/Ice Rescue
- ☐ Wildland Fire Fighter 1
- ☐ Wildland Fire Fighter 2

Signature:_____

Copyright 2000, Performance Training Systems, Inc.

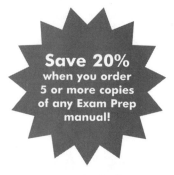